NO LONGER PROPERTY
OF ANYTHINK
RANGEVIEW LIBRARY
DISTRICT

D0828478

Praise for *The Yass Method for Pain-Free Movement*

"Dr. Yass's insights can help relieve the suffering of chronic pain for millions. His observation that most bodily pain results from muscular imbalance is right on target, and his individualized approach to focused muscle strengthening is a major advance that really works."

— **Leo Galland**, M.D., author of *The Allergy Solution*

"Mitchell Yass has developed a proven system to reduce, and even eliminate, chronic pain. If you've been told you just have to live with it, the wonderful and inspiring news is that you don't."

— **Bryan Hubbard**, publisher, *What Doctors Don't Tell You*

The Yass
METHOD
for Pain-Free
Movement

ALSO BY DR. MITCHELL YASS

The Pain Cure Rx:
The Yass Method for Diagnosing and Resolving Chronic Pain

Overpower Pain:
The Strength-Training Program That Stops Pain without Drugs or Surgery

All of the above are available at your local bookstore, or may be ordered by visiting:

Hay House USA: www.hayhouse.com
Hay House Australia: www.hayhouse.com.au
Hay House UK: www.hayhouse.co.uk
Hay House India: www.hayhouse.co.in

DR. MITCHELL YASS

The Yass METHOD
for Pain-Free Movement

A Guide to Easing through Your Day
without Aches and Pains

HAY HOUSE, INC.
Carlsbad, California • New York City
London • Sydney • Johannesburg • New Delhi

Copyright © 2018 by Mitchell Yass

Published in the United States by: Hay House, Inc.: www.hayhouse.com® • **Published in Australia by:** Hay House Australia Pty. Ltd.: www.hayhouse.com.au • **Published in the United Kingdom by:** Hay House UK, Ltd.: www.hayhouse.co.uk • **Published in India by:** Hay House Publishers India: www.hayhouse.co.in

Indexer: Jay Kreider
Illustrations by: Scott Leighton, provided by Dr. Mitchell Yass
Photos by: Dr. Mitchell Yass, Lisa Yass and Natalya Yass

All rights reserved. No part of this book may be reproduced by any mechanical, photographic, or electronic process, or in the form of a phonographic recording; nor may it be stored in a retrieval system, transmitted, or otherwise be copied for public or private use—other than for "fair use" as brief quotations embodied in articles and reviews—without prior written permission of the publisher.

The author of this book does not dispense medical advice or prescribe the use of any technique as a form of treatment for physical, emotional, or medical problems without the advice of a physician, either directly or indirectly. The intent of the author is only to offer information of a general nature to help you in your quest for emotional, physical, and spiritual well-being. In the event you use any of the information in this book for yourself, the author and the publisher assume no responsibility for your actions.

Library of Congress Cataloging-in-Publication Data

Names: Yass, Mitchell T, 1961- author.
Title: The Yass method for pain-free movement : a guide to easing through
   your day without aches and pains / Dr. Mitchell Yass.
Description: Carlsbad, California : Hay House, Inc., [2018]
Identifiers: LCCN 2017060612 | ISBN 9781401954611 (hardback)
Subjects: LCSH: Chronic pain--Exercise therapy. | Muscle strength. |
   Exercise--Physiological aspects. | Self-care, Health. | BISAC: HEALTH &
   FITNESS / Pain Management. | MEDICAL / Allied Health Services / Physical
   Therapy. | HEALTH & FITNESS / Healing.
Classification: LCC RB127 .Y38 2018 | DDC 616/.0472--dc23 LC record available at
   https://lccn.loc.gov/2017060612

Hardcover ISBN: 978-1-4019-5461-1

10 9 8 7 6 5 4 3 2 1
1st edition, May 2018

Printed in the United States of America

SUSTAINABLE
FORESTRY
INITIATIVE

Certified Chain of Custody
Promoting Sustainable Forestry
www.sfiprogram.org
SFI-01268

SFI label applies to the text stock

To my wife, Lisa, and my daughter, Natalya, thank you for your support during this difficult journey. Trying to exist without a safety net has been very difficult, but your love and affection have made it much easier. I love you both for allowing me to be who I think I need to be.

Contents

Introduction

Over the past quarter of a century, I have been addressing the issue of chronic pain with thousands of people who have suffered from months to decades. Chronic pain has become an acceptable condition in society worldwide, similar to a systemic disease such as cancer or cardiovascular disease. However, chronic pain is actually a cultural phenomenon and not a medical one. This line of thinking has been brought on by the advent of the MRI (magnetic resonance imaging) procedure, which finds structural variations like herniated discs, stenosis, pinched nerves, arthritis, meniscal tears, and the like and asserts that since these structural variations are identified at the time of pain, they must be the cause of pain. No logic, no theoretical basis, no multiyear study to show the correlation. It was simply unveiled and implemented. This is the primary explanation for the cause of chronic pain according to the medical establishment.

Pain is an indication of a tissue in distress. Pain is part of the body's defense mechanism. It is designed to provide a way for a tissue that is not functioning properly to create awareness of its failings so an intervention can be triggered to correct the issue. Quite simply, once the tissue is not functioning properly, acute pain is emitted. If the right tissue is identified and treated, the emergency distress call will no longer be needed and the pain will cease.

DISCOVERING THE TRUE SOURCE OF PAIN

From the time I entered medical school, I knew something was wrong with the existing academic curriculum when it came to the issue of diagnosing and treating pain. I decided to devise a method to identify the correct tissue that is in distress and thereby lead to the right treatment. This passion to find out how pain actually works became my focus morning, noon, and night. This was the intellectual aspect of the battle.

The emotional aspect of the battle came from treating thousands in which pain overtook their lives. I have treated patients who were suicidal, addicted to pain medication, depressed, despondent, or unable to maintain family relationships, a job, or to have a clear thought without pain overtaking their stream of consciousness. These were people pleading for help. They were willing to do anything to resolve their pain and get their lives back. They were angry and frustrated. They had done everything they were told to do and yet they still lived in pain. This emotional pain has been the primary driving force in my quest to create awareness of the true source of physical pain and its remedy.

One of the overriding questions that patients have when they hear about the Yass Method and its core principles is, "How come nobody else is doing this?" There is nothing more satisfying to me than seeing the transference of knowledge about the Yass Method to a person who has the potential to now have power over their body and understand what they need to do to resolve their pain and, better yet, to prevent it from recurring. This was never just a job for me. It started off being a quest for knowledge and ended up being a quest to end the plague of chronic pain worldwide.

What you must understand is that chronic pain is *not* the result of chronic disease. Chronic pain is the result of misdiagnosed acute pain. Chronic pain should not be perceived like a disease. Instead, it is part of the body's protective mechanism. It is not its own entity like a tissue. You don't treat pain. You treat the tissue in distress that is eliciting pain. To achieve this, you need to properly diagnose that tissue. You need the Yass Method. The problem with the existing system is not that it doesn't know how to treat pain. The problem is that it doesn't know how to diagnose the tissue in distress eliciting pain.

RESOLVING CHRONIC PAIN WITH THE YASS METHOD

Over two decades of my career, I've looked for common links among the thousands of patients I've treated for chronic pain. Was there something tangible that presented as a uniform among those suffering from chronic pain? Was there a way to isolate these trouble sources to prevent them from ever recurring? It quickly became clear that those suffering from chronic pain seemed to describe their pain in connection to performing functional activities in their daily lives. They would note the pain would come if they climbed stairs, tried to kneel, sat for a period of time, reached up, reached behind, or walked extensively. For some the pain would occur when performing the activity, while for others, the pain came afterward. There was no question, however, that if they did nothing, the pain wouldn't occur. This, naturally, led me to associate the pain with dysfunction. And I realized that the tissue associated with the dysfunction was muscle.

Because of my personal background in weight lifting and understanding the mechanics of the body, I was able to differentiate which muscles were associated with the particular activity/activities that would lead my patients to experience pain. The amazing part was that the body was also presenting symptoms such as altered posture, pain elicited in a muscle, weakness and flexibility deficits, and altered movement patterns that helped me confirm that I was correct in identifying the offending muscles. It became apparent that muscle was the offending tissue in almost every case that I treated. I wanted to take my understanding further and try to derive a theory as to why muscles were breaking down and preventing function from occurring without symptoms being developed.

And it finally hit me: *gravity!* We live in a gravity environment, which means that any activity, barring lying flat on the floor, will have a vertical force applied to us. For any activity to be performed, we are going to have to apply forces equal to or greater than that of gravity using our muscles or they will break down and generate symptoms of pain. This one deceptively simple principle actually explains everything. The shocking aspect to the theory is that it even answers why people get structural variations such as arthritis, herniated discs, stenosis, and similar variations.

My last book, *The Pain Cure Rx*, focused on pinpointing the origin of your pain (the tissue eliciting the symptom) and where those agonizing symptoms came from. In more than 95 percent of cases that I have treated, the cause was muscular, so I provided simple exercises to rebuild muscles that were clearly in distress, impeding your productivity, or forcing you to give up the activities you enjoyed.

Beyond the discussion of which tissue was creating the person's symptoms, I always found myself trying to simplify my unique and original theory about why people have pain in the first place. I truly felt that this was a key for people to understand if they were to make the Yass Method more than just a way of resolving pain. It was an attempt to empower them to be able to make better decisions about how they would be treated in the future. I wanted to make them understand that in most cases the cause of pain is mechanical—not structural, as most medical practitioners seem to incorrectly emphasize.

In order to perform the activities we do daily, we need to make gravity our friend. We must align and rebuild our muscles. In the majority of cases of pain, either a muscle strains and elicits pain or a muscle strains and causes another muscle to have to compensate, which in turn causes that muscle to strain. Or alternately a muscle may strain and create a symptom in another location (something most people are not even aware can occur), or else a muscle strains and impinges on a nearby nerve, causing irritation of the nerve leading it to create a symptom in another location (which is the case with sciatica). Regardless of the source of your symptoms, finding a way for your muscles to mitigate the forces of gravity will allow you to perform the functional tasks and activities that comprise your daily life.

My goal for this book is to support you through the activities that make up your life, to empower you with knowledge and ensure that you find the solutions you seek to live a better and pain-free life. I want to show you how to build the strength and dexterity to perform your daily activities to the fullest functional level without pain.

The Yass Method for Pain-Free Movement is not about undergoing multiple consultations with specialists, myself included, to get your results. It's about learning and employing a method of living that gives you the freedom and permission you need to return to a life of enjoyment, productivity, and physical ease throughout your day.

It's time to learn how to get pain-free movement through the Yass Method, so let's get started!

CHAPTER ONE

The Why of Your Pain

As part of my professional career in treating the issue of chronic pain, I have focused on formulating a theory as to why people suffer from pain. By understanding the reason that people suffer from pain, I believe it not only makes it easier to resolve pain, but to prevent it from even occurring. My educational background was in medical school in the physical therapy program. It was there that I immediately recognized a lack of logic and theoretical basis for what was being identified as the cause of pain regardless of where the pain was in the body. The emphasis on structure as the cause of pain was primarily derived from the use of the MRI as the mechanism for diagnosing its cause. Within a year of my graduating and beginning to practice as a physical therapist, the first MRI study was performed on people with no lower back pain. The 1994 study found that almost three quarters of people with no back pain had bulging or herniated discs.[1] This reinforced my theory that structural variations, in fact, were not the cause of pain for most people.

From the very earliest part of my training, the vast majority of people I encountered who were suffering from chronic pain seemed to have a muscular cause for the pain. This was even when they were diagnosed with a structural cause from an MRI. Once I recognized the muscular cause, I needed to understand why. It dawned on me that muscle is the primary tissue responsible for function, and most people seem to associate their pain with a particular activity they would perform. Whether the pain was experienced at the time of the activity or after, there was no question that performing that activity incited the pain. It was this connection between the inability to perform functional activities and the resulting development of pain that allowed me to create my theoretical basis for the Yass Method.

Most people suffer from pain because the muscles responsible for performing activities throughout the day are not strong enough to do so. This leads to the muscles straining and emitting pain. It can also cause the muscles to weaken or become unbalanced, thereby creating a misalignment of joint surfaces. *The functional activity loads for every person are different, so it is a matter of figuring out the relationship between the strengths of the muscles of the person versus the strength requirements of the activities being performed.*

If you are very sedentary, then you don't require as much muscle strength as someone who is performing more strenuous activity. This is not to say that a very active person can't have pain; it simply means that because of the greater force requirements of their activities, the muscles required for the activities must be stronger. Clearly the person who is sedentary doesn't use their muscles a lot. If they are suddenly called upon to perform some activity like climbing stairs or standing for a period of time, they are more susceptible to straining and having pain than the person who is more active and fit and whose muscles would be prepared to perform these activities without the chance of straining.

I have treated so many people who tell me they don't understand why they are experiencing pain in their later years after decades of living an active and painless life. I always try to make them understand that pain in the present has nothing to do with their previous abilities. Simply put, if the force requirement of activities today is greater than the force output of the muscles involved, the muscles will strain and pain will be the result.

Groups of muscles create functional activities. So if all but one muscle is strong enough to perform an activity, this will still cause the rest of the muscles to take the load of the weakened muscle, which is a load they were not designed to absorb. This will lead to other muscles straining and emitting pain. All muscles must be strong to allow for functional capacity without painful symptoms. Therefore, a full understanding of how to strengthen all the individual muscles necessary for function is a foundational component of the Yass Method.

There is a major lack of understanding as to what actually constitutes proper exercise. For instance, there is a culturally accepted idea that walking is an excellent form of exercise to help strengthen muscles. This is simply a fallacy. If you try to walk and a particular muscle is weak, your body simply alters how you walk and causes other muscles to compensate. Over time this leads muscles to take loads they were not designed to take. All the other forms of exercise, including bicycling, water aerobics, Pilates, and yoga, fall under the same category that uses multiple muscles to perform them. The only form of exercise that allows for individual muscles to be isolated and strengthened is targeted progressive strength training, which is a bedrock principle of the Yass Method.

One major culprit for the continuation of preventable pain is the medical establishment's use of the MRI to identify the cause of pain. The theory has been that since the MRI finds structural variations at the time a person is experiencing pain, this means that the structural variation found must be the cause of the pain. There is also the culturally induced belief that these structural variations should be perceived like cancers and as such require an immediate intervention upon their identification. The evidence, however, is overwhelmingly clear that in most cases these structural variations existed for years or even decades before the pain began, and therefore it is impossible to assert with certainty that structural variations are the cause of painful symptoms simply because they are identified in connection to an individual's pain.

This naturally provokes a major question: If structural causes found on MRIs like herniated discs, stenosis, and arthritis are not the cause of pain, then what accounts for these variations being found on diagnostic tests in so many people? My answer is that the cause of these structural variations is actually precipitated by the same source of pain. Just as a lack of strength or muscle imbalance can cause muscles to strain and elicit pain, these imbalances can also cause the misalignment of joint surfaces. When the surface area of joints decreases, this impedes the joint's ability to take the full force of a movement, which can then lead to deterioration of structural components. So arthritis, stenosis, herniated discs, and meniscal tears are actually, in most cases, the result of muscle weakness or imbalance. The fact that structural variations are so often found to be the cause of pain rather than the degenerative result of muscle weakness or imbalance is a major and potentially dangerous flaw in the pervasive methodology for diagnosing chronic pain.

THE BACK STORY

Since 1994, when the first MRI studies were performed on people with absolutely no back pain, the ability of the MRI to identify the cause of pain has been in question. As I mentioned at the beginning of the chapter, that 1994 study revealed that roughly 70 percent of people with no back pain could still be found to have herniated or bulging discs.[2] Likewise, another study showed that of those over the age of 60, 90 percent of people with no back pain were found to have bulging or degenerative discs.[3] In 2007, the American College of Physicians recommended that MRIs no longer be used to identify the cause of lower back pain because a 20-year literature search determined that in more than 85 percent of cases, the cause of the lower back pain could not be attributed to a spinal abnormality, such as a herniated disc or stenosis.[4] In 2005, neurosurgeon Dr. Aaron Filler created the MRN (magnetic resonance neurography), which is a higher-powered MRI able to identify nerves in tissue rather than only the spinal cord and nerve roots. Dr. Filler's study determined that in 93 percent of cases of sciatica, the cause was the sciatic nerve being impinged by a muscle in the gluteal region called the piriformis.[5]

The cause, then, had nothing to do with the lumbar spine or any structural variations like a herniated disc or stenosis. Studies on surgeries of structural abnormalities found on X-rays and MRIs have shown no better ability to decrease pain than mock surgeries. The medical establishment consequently created a new diagnosis—"failed back surgery syndrome"—to account for all those getting back surgery and still having the same if not greater pain after the surgery.[6] The reality is that in most cases the MRI finds structural abnormalities that are degenerative in nature, taking years to progress and never emitting a pain signal. It is incapable of identifying any muscular cause of pain, such as a muscle spasm, muscle strain, muscle imbalance, or lack of flexibility. The fact that it finds certain structural variations that can be found in almost as many people without pain as those with pain should provide enough evidence that it is time to end its use as the primary method in identifying the cause of pain.

HOW IS THE YASS METHOD DIFFERENT?

The Yass Method creates awareness of the cause of pain by using the exact system that the body has designed for that purpose. It provides a set of symptoms that, when interpreted, tell you which tissue is the cause of the pain. However, the goal of this system is to focus on the cause, rather than only the symptoms themselves. When you do that, you get to the root of your problem. And when you get to the root of the problem, you have a clear opportunity to resolve your pain.

Most people would agree that if they had pain in their chest and left arm, they wouldn't ignore these symptoms due to a general understanding that these symptoms represent a very specific cause: a heart attack. The neck, the back, and the extremities work exactly the same way. Depending on the particular tissue that is in distress and responsible for the symptoms being created, the particular symptoms being experienced represent a very specific cause of tissue in distress. The idea that pain is somehow nondescript and requires a diagnostic test to identify which tissue is in distress is a fallacy. The most common tissues associated with pain in the extremities, neck, and back are muscle, nerve, and bone. Each one of these areas presents with specific symptoms that can indicate which tissue is creating the pain.

For example, let's say you have pain at the shoulder. If the cause was a muscle strain, you would have difficulty moving your shoulder through a range of motion because the muscles that are strained would inhibit that and cause pain. Now let's say another person tried to move your shoulder through the same motion. There should be no problem doing so because the muscles are not being used in this case. In the Yass Method, this would indicate that the cause is muscular. Alternately, if arthritis were the cause of the pain, then you would expect there to be a loss of range of motion, whether the person in pain moved the shoulder or somebody moved the shoulder for them. This is because arthritis would develop in the joint and inhibit motion of the shoulder, regardless of who moved it.

Fig. 1-1a. Active testing of range of motion of the shoulder joint	**Fig. 1-1b. Passive testing of range of motion of the shoulder joint**
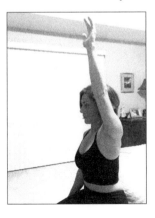	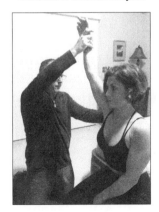

This illustrates one of the primary principles of the Yass Method, which is to first determine if the cause of pain is structural or muscular. If structural, no amount of strengthening will resolve the cause. In most of these cases, only surgery will work. Conversely, if the cause is muscular, no amount of surgery will resolve the symptoms. Only targeting and strengthening the correct muscles will alleviate the pain. Thus, surgery, even as a last resort, is completely illogical. If the cause is indeed muscular, then surgery should not be an option at all, regardless of other unsuccessful treatments.

If a structural abnormality is the cause of pain at a peripheral joint, it will cause a loss of range of motion and will at a certain point feel like a bone is hitting another bone, further limiting the motion. Pain is an indication of a tissue in distress; therefore, if the full range of motion is intact, there is no reason to think that pain is being caused by the structure of the joint. Counter to the medical diagnostic methodology, the Yass Method considers how the body tries to create awareness of a tissue in distress by eliciting very specific symptoms of pain from that tissue.

For example, when MRIs find a rotator cuff tear, the pain at the shoulder region is immediately associated with the MRI finding. The problem with this is that the identified tear most likely is degenerative. If an MRI were taken before the pain occurred, the tear would have been identified. Reality must meet what is seen. In almost every case I have treated where the diagnosis through an MRI was a rotator cuff tear, the person had a nearly full range of motion of the shoulder. With a true rotator cuff tear, range of motion would be severely decreased. If the tear were the cause of the pain, then a specific incident would have to be identified as the cause of the tear, designated by a full range of motion before the incident and a major loss after. There would have to have been no pain before and then pain after the incident. In almost every case I've ever treated, the rotator cuff strain occurred with other muscles straining as well. The presentation of the symptoms—including the location of the pain, what types of movements bring on the symptoms, and how the shoulder and shoulder blade act when the person moves their shoulder—are all contributing indicators of understanding the cause of the pain. In this case, the cause is most likely to be a rotator cuff strain.

SO WHAT IS THE CAUSE OF PAIN?

As far as I know, I am the only person to ever create a theoretical basis of why people have pain. In most cases, this is not even a consideration within the medical establishment. In fact, the failure to properly identify and treat the cause of pain has led to a flourishing cottage industry of various outrageous theories and practices. There are those who now think that pain is being elicited from the brain for no reason, which has in turn led to a whole movement toward altering the brain's perception of real, stimulus-caused pain through meditation and drugs. Then there are those promoting an interpretation of pain as "inflammation." So the Western medicine folks promote lots of drugs to address the so-called inflammation, while the Eastern medicine folks promote herbs and other "natural" remedies. The problem here is that for *inflammation* to be present where pain is being experienced, the body would present specific symptoms, including *swelling, heat,* and *redness, along with specific sorts of pain.* In my experience, I have found this in less than one-tenth of one percent of the population. (When the symptoms were present, I did address the pain as being related to inflammation and tried to designate a specific cause.)

Then there are the folks who think the pain is not physical at all. They theorize that pain is from a repressed emotion pent up for years and that the emotional disturbances present pain at the neck, the back, or an extremity. My problem with this theory is that the physical presentation of the symptoms often show a specific tissue eliciting the symptoms and, in the case of muscle, indicate a clear muscular deficit. While emotional distress is certainly a non-negligible component to our experience of physical pain, I would argue that the emotional aspect comes from being unable to properly diagnose and treat the true cause of the pain. A smaller sect believes that pain is due to a bad diet and lack of appropriate nutrients, which similarly fails to account for muscular strain and degenerative causes. The very sad reality is that because of the completely baseless means of using MRIs or other diagnostic tests to identify the cause of pain, all of these somewhat irrational ideas have festered, leaving those suffering with chronic pain to reach for the unproven and illogical.

The key to determining which tissue is the cause of the pain is through the evaluative techniques incorporated in the Yass Method.

IS THE YASS METHOD FOR EVERYONE?

If the evaluative techniques indicate that the cause of the pain is muscular, then the only answer to resolving that pain is targeted strength training. If the techniques indicate that the cause of the pain is structural, like a herniated disc, stenosis, meniscal tear, or arthritis, then all the strength training in the world will not resolve the cause. I would be for surgery in these cases as soon as possible, with post-surgery physical therapy to address the postsurgical symptoms and confirm that full strength and balance of all muscle is achieved in order to prevent future symptoms. The Yass Method is designed to prevent the misapplication of exercise and surgical treatment by identifying the underlying cause of chronic pain. If the cause is structural, surgery is the only solution. If the cause of pain is muscular, then targeted strength training is the only solution.

Ultimately, as a medical practitioner, I have one goal and that is to resolve the cause of pain in order to allow my patients to lead the most fulfilling lives possible. After more than two decades of watching people suffer needlessly for years on end, I am very humbled and honored that so many have felt compelled to reach out to me to help return them to the lives they have lost for so long.

For those who have had surgery and are still suffering with pain, I am very happy to inform you that the Yass Method will still work for you. If the cause was muscular before the surgery, that means the cause will still be muscular, which means that targeted strength training can be used to resolve the cause of the pain. My goal is to identify the cause as muscular before an unnecessary surgery is performed, which can exacerbate the lack of muscle use in the area of the surgery, further impeding the muscles from obtaining the strength they need to resolve the pain and return to full function. So if you underwent a surgery that did nothing to reduce your symptoms, or may have even increased them, take solace in knowing that you can still resolve your pain and get back to the life you deserve. For people who had surgery and are still experiencing the same presurgery symptoms, it is likely that the wrong tissue was treated, which should incite hope because if the right tissue is identified and treated, the symptoms will cease.

EXERCISING THE MUSCLE

When it comes to identifying the cause of muscular pain, you must understand which muscles work to either stabilize a joint or move a joint to allow a functional task to be performed. There are specific muscle tests that can be utilized to determine which muscles have been strained and which muscles need to be strengthened or lengthened (these tests will be discussed in the subsequent chapters). It is this understanding that allows you to know specifically which muscles must be worked on to achieve balance in the muscular system, which will in turn allow function to occur without symptoms. The strengthening needed to resolve pain is targeted in that you only want to strengthen the affected muscles. While fitness experts might promote the notion that strengthening all muscles is the way to go, overall exercise routines will not resolve the symptoms elicited by a specific tissue or muscular deficit. In fact, overstrengthening non-distressed muscles may worsen your symptoms.

Let's say, for example, that you have knee pain and it is because your front thigh muscles—the quadriceps, or quads—have become too strong in relation to the posterior thigh muscles, the hamstrings. This could cause the quads to shorten and consequently pull excessively on the kneecap, causing it to become excessively compressed in the knee joint when the knee is bent and straightened, leading to pain at the knee joint. The standard theory of general strengthening would have this person strengthening both the quads and hamstrings and, from my understanding of how people strengthen, would most likely be aggressive in strengthening the quads because that is a very common thing to do. In strengthening both the hamstrings and quads, you would be sustaining the very imbalance that has led to the pain, and therefore would do nothing to correct the muscular deficit responsible for the knee pain.

Let's play out another classic example of a lack of understanding of how to precisely strengthen the required muscles versus the use of a general strengthening attitude. A person is thought to have strained their rotator cuff. They are directed to strengthen the shoulder region in the hope of resolving the pain associated with the strained rotator cuff. A typical strategy for this condition is to develop improved internal and external rotation, because it is generally understood that the rotator cuff is connected to these motions of the shoulder.

INTERNAL ROTATION

Fig. 1-2a. Start of internal rotation

Fig. 1-2b. End of internal rotation

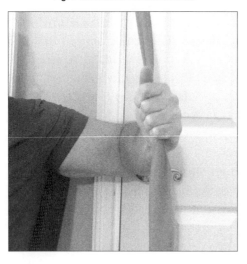

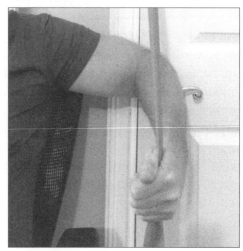

EXTERNAL ROTATION

Fig. 1-2c. Start of external rotation

Fig. 1-2d. End of external rotation

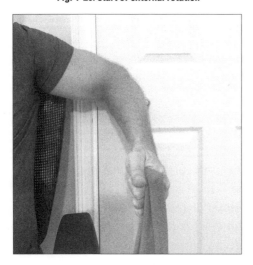

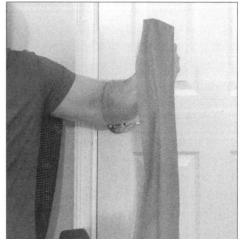

Here is the problem with this scenario. All muscles create their optimal force at their optimal length. In the case of a strained muscle, the length of the muscle after the strain must be determined to see if the strain was mild and the muscle is still at the optimal length or whether the strain was more severe and now the muscle has shortened. If the muscle has shortened and you try to strengthen it, it will have a tendency to get shorter, meaning you are actually impeding the muscle from achieving its optimal length and optimal force. In the case of the rotator cuff, a flexibility test must be performed to determine its length. The rotator cuff should be able to be stretched to 90 degrees of motion from its original position. If it is less than 90 degrees, then this muscle cannot be strengthened at this time.

Fig. 1-3a. 90 degrees internal rotation

Fig. 1-3b. Short of 90 degrees internal rotation

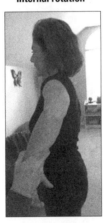 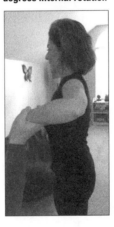

In fact, the opposite must occur. The muscles that oppose the rotator cuff must be strengthened to help lengthen the muscle to its optimal length to allow for normal pain-free shoulder function. If you took the path of general strengthening as being a good way to go, you would be performing both internal and external rotation from the initial start of addressing the strain, and the length of the muscle would be forever unchanged, continuing to strain and elicit pain at the shoulder region.

This flaw in understanding muscles and how muscles work is systemic. There is no medical specialty with the educational or training experience to provide a proper understanding to lead to successful outcomes. The fitness industry is also devoid of this level of comprehension. So my suggestion to all those suffering who in fact have muscular deficits is to learn exactly which muscles are responsible for your symptoms so the right muscles can be strengthened with the correct exercises.

Another key point in the Yass Method is resistance. *Resistance is the only mechanism that will allow a muscle to become stronger.* Repetition will not do it. Performing an exercise just by actively moving a joint will not succeed in strengthening a muscle. So knowing how to correctly use resistance to work against a muscle and make it stronger is another integral component to targeted strength training. This leads to the resolution of symptoms and return to full functional capacity in the shortest period of time for old and young people alike.

The primary reason that most prescribed medical or fitness programs fail to resolve muscular causes of symptoms is due to a lack of understanding about the importance of resistance. I would say that the vast majority of people I've treated whose previous treatments failed told me that they simply performed exercises without any resistance or very benign levels of resistance. This may be due in part to a misguided key cornerstone of the physical therapy establishment, which asserts that practitioners should never try to strengthen a muscle until the pain is resolved, meaning that if the cause of pain is muscular and requires targeted progressive resistance strength training to resolve the cause, conventional physical therapy may well fail to address it.

When talking about incorporating some form of exercise to resolve the cause of pain when the cause is found to be muscular, there is a lot of misinformation that may lead people away from utilizing progressive resistance. The medical establishment often promotes yoga, walking, bicycling, or other forms of fitness activities as the way to strengthen deficits. The fundamental problem with this is that these activities require multiple muscles to perform, and will consequently fail to isolate the distressed muscles in need of strengthening. In fact, the body's tendency will be to overcompensate and make other muscles work harder until they strain too. The false premise in promoting these activities as being valid mechanisms to resolve pain due to muscular deficits is the false premise that the more time you spend exercising will make you stronger and somehow address the specific muscular deficits leading to your symptoms. This is completely invalid.

Time is not a factor in getting specific muscles stronger. Likewise, the idea of more is better is actually the opposite of what is true. When properly performing a progressive resistance strength-training program, actively strengthening a distressed muscle more than three times weekly is detrimental and more apt to cause the muscle to strain. By using progressive resistance to strengthen muscles, the muscle is actually broken down through a process of creating muscular microtears. The 24- to 48-hour period after a strength-training activity allows the body and the targeted muscle to heal. Therefore, you would not want to try to strengthen during this period of time, as the muscle is more susceptible to straining during the healing process. This is why I never have any individual I work with strengthen any particular muscle more than three times a week.

So with the understanding that time is not the factor in healing and getting stronger, the next question becomes (well, even if you have figured out that you need to perform isolated strength-training exercises for the appropriate muscles), how many repetitions is the right number? The conventional recommendation with repetitions is to start off performing 10 repetitions, and then when it gets easier, go to 12 or 15 and eventually up to 20 repetitions. But this will actually *prevent* you from getting stronger.

When a muscle contracts, lactic acid begins to build up. Lactic acid actually impedes the ability of a muscle to contract. So as time goes by and you progress to higher repetitions of an exercise, lactic acid is causing less muscle mass to be available to perform the exercise. As you get into 15 or 20 repetitions in a set, maybe 50 to 60 percent of all the muscle mass is available. So the exercise feels harder, not because all of your muscle could not move the resistance being applied, but because you simply have less muscle mass to move the resistance. If you accept the idea that strength training is intended to make the most amount of muscle mass move the most amount of resistance, then the use of higher repetitions in sets of exercise prevents this from being obtainable. I never have any person I work with do more than 10 repetitions in a set for this reason. It is also one of the reasons why the people I work with get stronger the fastest and see the results of decreased symptoms and increased functional capacity in the quickest time frame available.

So if how often you exercise is not the key to obtaining maximal strength in the shortest period of time and doing more repetitions is not going to achieve this goal, then what is? ***The answer is simply increasing the resistance of the exercises performed in the shortest period of time.*** The exercises being performed are simply mechanisms and will do nothing to resolve your symptoms on their own merit alone. It is the application of progressive resistance to thoughtful exercises that will achieve the goal of full resolution of symptoms and full functional capacity.

Another key point completely missing from the understanding of how to maximize strength training is knowing how long you should wait between sets of exercise being performed before doing the next set. There are many who think that limiting the time between sets is beneficial and helps to make muscles stronger. This again goes completely against logic. As I mentioned before, as a muscle contracts, lactic acid naturally develops and limits the ability of a muscle to contract. In fact, a muscle that cramps is usually one that is perfuse with lactic acid to the point where the muscle becomes incapable of contracting. When the muscle is contracting, the microcirculation that runs through the muscle is compressed with blood not able to run through the muscle. Once the exercise ends and the muscle is resting, the microcirculation opens and blood can enter the muscle and remove the lactic acid. The intensity of the bout of exercise will determine how much lactic acid has developed and how much time it will take for it to be removed from the muscle in order for the full muscle mass to be available to perform the next exercise set.

Generally I have found that about a one-minute rest is the appropriate time frame between sets. A simple way to know if you have waited long enough can be seen in the following example. You just completed a set of 10 repetitions with a set resistance. You did not wait long enough for all the lactic acid to be removed from the muscle and you try the next set in which you only get 8 repetitions with the same resistance. It isn't possible that you somehow lack the same amount of muscle mass as the first set in which you were able to perform 10 repetitions with the set resistance. What happened was that you just didn't have 100 percent of that muscle mass for the second set because you didn't wait long enough in between the sets. Without having 100 percent of your muscle mass for each set, you limit your ability to adapt to the maximal amount of resistance, thereby limiting your ability to maximize your strength and achieve the pain-free functional lifestyle you are seeking in the shortest period of time.

In short, if the cause of your symptoms is muscle weakness or imbalance and you want to perform a progressive resistance strength-training program to resolve your symptoms and achieve a full functional lifestyle again, you need to:

- Identify which specific muscles are responsible for your symptoms
- Learn which exercises are recommended for addressing the muscular deficits and how to perform them correctly

- Never attempt to strengthen any muscle more than three times a week, and never do more than 10 repetitions in a set

- Progress the resistance you are using in the shortest time frame possible

- Perform the sets with about a one-minute break between sets

INTRODUCTION TO STRENGTHENING YOUR MUSCLES

Many of you have been taught how to exercise from traditional medical practitioners or personal trainers, and a certain amount of deprogramming will likely be required here. There are many misnomers that are represented regarding the proper way to perform exercise or to "strengthen" a muscle, which can inhibit people from achieving the goal of strengthening their muscles. You will need to understand how to isolate a muscle while stabilizing the rest of your body to utilize the maximum amount of energy available for your muscle to work against the maximum resistance. You will learn about the use of progressive resistance to cause a muscle to get stronger. You will learn about all the possible inhibitors of using the maximal amount of strength of a muscle in performing a strength-training exercise, such as not waiting long enough between sets, doing too many repetitions in a set, and not being fully stabilized when performing the exercise. The Yass Method of strengthening incorporates an all-inclusive body of information to isolate the appropriate muscles and strengthen them in the shortest period of time. As with any strength-training program, before performing the Yass Method exercises, you need to understand some very basic concepts. By the time I am finished with this section, I hope you have a clear understanding of why you are being asked to perform the exercises in the specific Yass Method manner, as well as how to do them correctly and efficiently. The recommended exercises will be presented throughout the chapters where specific strength-training remedies are identified as well as at the end of the book in the Appendix.

WHAT DOES IT MEAN TO ISOLATE A MUSCLE?

The two primary components of the Yass Method exercise regimen are *isolating* the correct muscle with the proper exercise and *strengthening* the isolated muscle with progressive resistance so that it gets stronger and increases its mass.

Let's start with the first idea of isolating the correct muscle. If you are performing an exercise where more than one muscle is working, the weakened muscle will not be isolated. The other muscles will pick up the slack to take the stress off the weakened muscle, which may continue to get weaker. Even worse, in allowing for the compensation to continue, other muscles will be overworked and they will begin to strain and cause symptoms. If you perform exercises that do not isolate a muscle so that it can be strengthened appropriately, you will not only fail to achieve the exercise's goal, but you will also stand a good chance of making things worse by straining other muscles.

Remember that exercises such as running on a treadmill, bicycling, yoga, and Pilates do not isolate a single muscle at a time. Muscles attach to joints and move a joint in a single place. For instance, the bicep (front upper arm) muscle bends the elbow, moving the hand toward shoulder with the palm facing up. The tricep (posterior upper arm) muscle extends, or straightens, the elbow. The quad muscle of the front thigh straightens the knee while the hamstrings, or posterior thigh muscle, bend the knee. You can see that each muscle is moving a joint in one direction or plane. If any exercise is asking for you to move more than one joint in a single direction or plane, then by definition you will not be isolating a specific muscle.

Now let's take this idea even further. If you are trying to isolate a weakened muscle, you will want to do everything in your power to avoid incorporating any other muscles into the exercise. You will want to put all your effort into having that one muscle work against the most amount of resistance it safely can. If you perform a bicep curl, you can do it in a standing or a sitting position. But which position best isolates the bicep so it pushes against the most amount of resistance? The sitting position would be better, because standing requires the muscles that support and balance you to contract. This will divert energy away from the bicep muscle. Sitting allows you to use more resistance with the bicep, getting it stronger faster. When possible, it is preferable to perform exercises while seated, which allows you to better isolate the muscle you are trying to strengthen.

WHAT CAUSES A MUSCLE TO GET STRONGER?

A muscle is composed of two proteins: actin and myosin. Each fiber of muscle consists of these two proteins. Actin looks like a line of balls all in a row. Myosin looks like a golf club with a shaft and a head. The way a muscle contracts is that the golf club head (myosin) will push a ball (actin) to the side until it is in line with the ball that is adjacent to it. The club head will then engage with this adjacent ball and push it over until it is in line with the next ball. This continues on as a process. Imagine now that there are a billion golf clubs pushing balls to the side until they are in line with the next ball and so forth, such that one protein slides along the other. As the golf club pushes the ball, force is created. This is how a muscle creates force. How strong a muscle is depends on how many golf clubs can engage balls. If you want to make a muscle stronger, you have to build muscle mass and make more golf clubs and balls.

Since a muscle works by creating force, causing the muscle to adapt to a greater force than it is used to creating will allow new muscle to grow. The only way a muscle can get stronger is by adapting to greater and greater resistances. Once it's stronger, activities will be performed without straining or eliciting symptoms.

Why is this understanding so important? Because there is so much bad information out there that this needs to be clarified. Most people will perform strengthening exercises doing a certain number of exercises for a particular muscle. They will perform a certain number of sets of the exercise and perform a certain number of repetitions per set. If the exercise becomes easier and they want to make the exercise more challenging, they will usually increase the number of repetitions or number of sets of the exercise. But if the resistance remains the same despite the number of sets or the number of repetitions increasing, there will be no incentive for the body to create more muscle mass. Therefore, you will not get stronger.

Let's be very clear here. The mechanism by which the resistance is developed doesn't matter. You can use dumbbells, barbells, machines, or even resistance bands and tubes. It only matters that the muscle is challenged appropriately to create force against a progressively increasing resistance.

FULL RANGE OF MOTION WITH A CONTROLLED SPEED

A muscle causes a joint to move in one plane through a set range of motion. When performing strength training, the goal is to cause the muscle to push a resistance through its joint's full range of motion. Why is this important? The resistance is only one factor in how the muscle adapts to the exercise. The distance that the resistance travels is the other. An effective exercise uses both factors to work the muscle against the most amount of resistance through a complete range of motion. Anything less than the full range of motion limits the total work that the muscle will perform and the ability of the muscle to adapt to the exercise.

Some people promote performing isometric contractions, defined as contractions of the muscle where no range of motion is being created. Others promote doing half the range of motion on one set and then the other half on another set. I am sure people can come up with multiple variables, but stick with the core principles of how to strengthen a muscle and you will get stronger the fastest.

While using resistance is key, it is important to do so responsibly. Just as I have had patients who were hesitant to increase the resistance they were using for fear of hurting themselves, I have had others who were so anxious to resolve their symptoms that they became very aggressive in trying to increase their resistance. The simplest way to know if you are using too much resistance is this: if you cannot complete the full range of motion of an exercise, then you are using too much resistance. The primary aspect of performing an exercise is completing the full range of motion. The amount of resistance used is secondary and is only appropriate if the full range of motion of the exercise is completed.

Next let's talk about how fast you should be moving. Moving too fast inhibits the muscle from pushing the resistance. But if you go too slow, lactic acid will develop at a quick rate and result in the loss of available muscle mass, limiting your ability to move the resistance. One of the worst rhythms is when resistance is jerked all over the place with the belief that the more momentum developed, the better. But the reality is that instead of the force output of your muscle, momentum will move the resistance. So, in fact, developing momentum inhibits the ability of a muscle to get stronger.

Doing an exercise with a controlled speed might not seem like much fun, but it is how the body works. Always remember that lactic acid development impedes the ability of a muscle to get stronger, and going too slowly when performing an exercise allows lactic acid to build up at a very fast pace. If it should take 10 seconds to perform a set with a certain resistance, you take 20 or 30 seconds, and you can't complete the full set of repetitions, it is because the amount of time for lactic acid to develop was so great that at the end there was no longer any muscle mass available to move the resistance. If you had performed the exercise with the same resistance in the proper time frame of 10 seconds, lactic acid would not have had enough time to develop. You should feel like the joint is moving at a comfortable speed while performing strength training. Momentum should never be developed, but do not prolong the time it takes to go through the range of motion either.

PROPER BREATHING

When performing the exercises, it is important to breathe properly, particularly as you use more strenuous resistances. Proper breathing helps to prevent you from holding your breath and building up pressure in the cardiovascular system. Also, when you exhale, you contract your abdominal muscles, which causes your torso and pelvis to be bonded together. This allows the muscles of the upper extremities or lower extremities to pull off their attachment to the torso or pelvis so that the muscles create more force and get stronger more easily. As a general rule, you want to exhale as the muscle is shortening and inhale as it is returning back to its normal length. If you are using free weights, such as dumbbells or barbells, exhale when moving against gravity and inhale when moving with gravity. If you are using resistance bands or tubes, exhale as the muscle shortens and inhale as it returns back to full length.

SETTING UP YOUR STRENGTH-TRAINING REGIMEN

I am guessing that most of you would say that you should be strength training every day. Remember, however, in reality, you should not be strengthening a muscle more than three times a week. I recommend performing the strength-training program either on a Monday, Wednesday, and Friday or Tuesday, Thursday, and Saturday.

Here's an important reminder on why a three-day-per-week program is most effective and safe: When you perform a strength-training program, you are actually breaking down muscle by creating microtears in it. This causes an inflammatory response to occur through which the body heals the muscle by making more muscle. This inflammatory response occurs for the next 24 to 48 hours after the bout of exercise is performed. Trying to strengthen during this period of time makes the muscle susceptible to straining and becoming injured. Thus, the exercise routine you perform should only be executed three times a week with a day in between the bouts of exercise for healing.

For each exercise, you should perform three sets of 10 repetitions with a one-minute rest between sets and exercises. For resistance, I would suggest using 50 percent of your maximal effort. In other words, if I asked you how difficult it is to perform a set of 10 repetitions with a certain weight on a scale of 1 to 10, where 1 feels like you are doing nothing and 10 feels like you might tear a muscle, you would want to start performing your exercise at a level of 5. Put another way, if I asked you whether you could have done 14 or 15 repetitions in the set, you would say you probably could have but that it would have been tough to achieve.

Once you feel you have a good sense of how to perform the exercises, you can move up to 80 percent of your maximal effort or an 8 on a scale of 1 to 10. This would feel like if I asked you if you could have done 11 or 12 repetitions, you would say you might have been able to but it would have been really tough to complete. I have found this to be the optimal exertion level for getting stronger while limiting the chance of injury.

Remember that the exercises being performed are only a mechanism to isolate weakened muscles and adapt them to greater resistances in order to allow you to perform functional activities without straining or eliciting symptoms. Regardless of how you create the resistance, whether through the use of weight-lifting machines, dumbbells, barbells, or resistance bands/tubes, the goal is always the same: start with an initial resistance of 50 percent and then progress to 80 percent of your maximal effort. Stick with this latter resistance level until the exertion level feels like 50 percent of the effort. This means that your muscles have adapted to this resistance and built muscle in response, causing the same resistance level to feel easier to perform.

Progression of Resistance through Exertion Scale

Start →	First progression →	Second progression →	Final progression
Resistance level: 5 out of 10.	Resistance level: 8 out of 10.	Resistance level: 5 out of 10.	Resistance level: 8 out of 10.
Feels like you can do 15 to 16 reps. Once you are comfortbable, go to first progression.	Feels like you can do 11 to 12 reps. Stay with this level of resistance until it feels like 5 out of 10.	Feels like you can do 15 to 16 reps. Once you are comfortable, go to the final progression.	Feels like you can do 11 to 12 reps. Stay with this level of resistance until it feels like 5 out of 10.

Once this occurs, increase the resistance so that the exertion returns to 80 percent of your maximal effort. Again, stick with this resistance level until your muscles adapt and the effort level feels like 50 percent of maximal effort, and so on and so forth. The goal of this process is to eventually develop enough strength that the force output of the muscles trying to perform a specific activity is greater than the force requirement of the activity. Once you reach that point, the activity will be performed with ease and without symptom. And once all activities are performed with ease and without symptom, you will have achieved your ultimate goal. At this point you can choose to sustain this level of resistance without the need to increase it. In the future, if you choose to perform an activity that requires more strength, then you can begin the progression of increasing resistances again to meet the needs of the more strenuous activity.

SAFE, NOT SORRY

Another aspect of trying to minimize lactic acid buildup in a muscle is the idea of stabilizing yourself when performing a strength-training exercise. There is limited thought about what is better—standing or sitting when doing the exercise—and yet this is a critical decision to help maximize your chances of getting stronger. If standing, you are asking your body to stabilize you while performing an exercise. This means that muscles beyond those moving the resistance must contract to create the balance and stability needed to perform the exercise. The risk here is that valuable energy that could be going toward the movement of the resistance in getting the specific muscle worked is being taken away and utilized by muscles needed for balance and stability. This is highly inefficient and limits your potential for success.

There has even been a push in the fitness world of the idea that more instability is better for performing exercises. People are being asked to perform single-legged exercises, to strengthen one arm while the other arm is statically holding a resistance, or to conduct exercises on stability balls and other unstable surfaces. Instability is something that can be effective when looking to improve balance usually associated with sports-specific activities, but it is extremely detrimental and ineffective when looking to strengthen an isolated muscle. Every time you divert energy from the working muscle to any muscle that is now required to enhance stability, you are moving away from achieving your goals. The best part of my targeted strength-training program is that most of the exercises are performed in the seated position, which more effectively allows you to isolate the muscle in need of strengthening.

Fig. 1-4a. Inefficient standing lat pulldown

Fig. 1-4b. Efficient seated lat pulldown

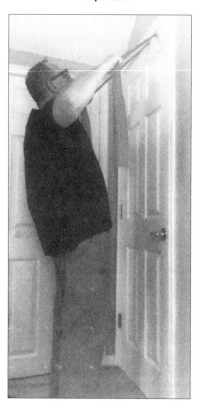
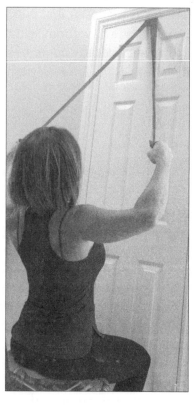

For many people, the idea of activity-induced pain being resolved through strength training seems counterintuitive. They often ask, "If I am having pain performing a functional activity, then how can I strength train and not have pain?" The answer lies in the fact that when you perform functional activities, you are using a lot of muscles to do so. If a muscle has strained enough to emit pain, this means other muscles must be compensating and overworking. As long as this situation exists, pain will be elicited with activity. But with my targeted strength training, most of the body is actually stable and only one muscle is working to perform the exercise. This prevents any other muscles from straining while performing the exercise. This is how you perform a strengthening exercise without experiencing pain. Once all of the muscles are adequately strengthened, they can work properly in performing tasks without eliciting pain. The last point to make here is that the word *resistance* should not be feared. Resistance can come in the form of a resistance band, free weights like dumbbells or barbells, or machines. The resistance can start off very mild and can over time be made more challenging. The key is to simply apply some form of resistance so the muscle is forced to get stronger and grow more muscle. This is the only way to make a muscle strong enough to perform tasks without breaking down.

THE FUTURE OF YOUR PAIN

By now you will see how revolutionary the Yass Method is in comparison to the conventional assumptions and attitudes within the medical and fitness establishments. I intend to make my method available to every person with unresolved pain, ultimately with the goal of elevating the Yass Method as a primary way of diagnosing and treating pain. There is no question that some people will require some medical assistance in resolving their pain, which is why we need a unified method of diagnosing and treating pain. Just as someone who has a heart problem goes to a cardiologist and expects a similar diagnostic and treatment protocol, this should hold true for pain. Everyone has the right to live without pain. I won't rest until every person is able to get the correct care they need.

With the understanding that 95 to 98 percent of cases of pain are muscular, I will now focus my attention on the different types of functional limitations you may be enduring over the course of your day. I will discuss the limiting functional activity or task, what is causing the limitation, and what is needed to resolve the limitation. Going forward in the book, things get very simple: locate the activity you are having trouble with, understand the cause of the difficulty, and correct the cause to eliminate this distraction and annoyance from your day. This is your chance to achieve *pain-free movement* in your life, now and for good!

CHAPTER TWO

Your Daily Life at Home

For most of us, life begins in the morning. The alarm clock goes off and leads us to the start of our day. For many this is the toughest time, when pain shows its ugly head with its greatest intensity.

Over the course of an active day, our muscles contract to perform activities or tasks. As a result, lactic acid develops. The lactic acid makes it more difficult for muscles to contract because it impedes the ability of the two proteins actin and myosin, which make up muscle, to grab one another, thereby creating force. The pH of the body can be affected by the development of the acidic material in lactic acid. The biochemical concern of the body is that if the blood becomes too acidic, this can be dangerous, so our bodies want to remove the lactic acid as a protective measure. Blood must enter the muscle to help wash the lactic acid from there to the liver, where it is reconstituted to become pyruvic acid, which can then be used to create energy for the body. Since blood is warm, the warmth of the blood running through the muscle can allow it to be maintained at a more lengthened position. Our pain receptors run on the connective tissue that surrounds the muscle fibers. Thus, the longer in length the muscle can be maintained, the more separated the pain receptors become and the less pain we experience.

Once you lie down to sleep, no activity is performed, meaning there is no lactic acid being developed in the muscles. Therefore, there is no reason for excessive blood to pass through the muscles, which means that the length of the muscles will be reduced while you sleep. Strained muscles in particular have a tendency to want to contract, leading to shortened muscles. As a result, when you wake up, your muscles are going to be the shortest that they will be throughout the day. Since the pain receptors run along the length of the muscles, this means that you'll likely experience the highest concentration of pain receptors along the muscles when you wake up after a night's sleep, and therefore why pain may be more intense at this time. A rational understanding of why you seem to have more pain when you first wake up will help you know how your body works and what steps you might take to resolve the pain.

Certainly the best long-term solution is to resolve any weakness or imbalance of muscle that can lead to straining and contracting when you wake up. In the short term, I have suggested to people that applying a heating pad to where the pain is being experienced is a way to prevent the muscles from shortening during the night. There are different types of menthol- or camphor-based adhesive pads that are known to provide three to four hours of warmth at a time. Some basic stretches before going to bed could also help to keep your muscles at their optimal length during the night, which is the key to limiting pain in the morning.

GOOD MORNING AND WAKING UP

Now that it is morning and you tried some of the suggestions I just described to maximize the length of your muscles before going to bed, if you are still having pain and an inability to move freely, this is your chance to perform a few more actions that will make the beginning of the day more pleasant and pain-free. Before starting the typical morning chores of brushing your teeth or combing your hair, I would suggest first taking a warm to hot shower. Those initial steps from the bed might be difficult, but once you are able to get into the shower and allow the warm/hot water to hit your body, especially in the areas where you are having pain, the increased temperature of the water will begin to increase blood flow throughout the body. Just like with the blood flow designed to get rid of lactic acid, the increased blood flow from the warm/hot water will allow your muscles to achieve a more lengthened position. This will cause the pain receptors that run along the length of the muscles to be separated and therefore decrease the level of pain being experienced.

Have you been told that the cause of your back pain was a herniated disc, stenosis, or pinched nerve? Or perhaps you were told that the cause of your peripheral joint pain was arthritis, a meniscal tear, or a labral tear. And yet when you take a hot shower in the morning, your pain seems to melt away. You now understand why. It was not the structural variation emitting the pain, but the muscle in the region. In taking the hot shower, you were lengthening the muscle and separating the pain receptors that run along the fibers. Be happy in knowing that the cause of your pain is actually muscular and that it can be fixed by steps you can take.

Now that you are feeling better after your warm/hot shower and you feel a bit more limber, let's take this to the next level. Let's perform a 15- to 20-minute stretching routine. This is not a lot of time, but it is time well spent. Once your muscles have been warmed up, you can now choose to be more aggressive in lengthening them further. One little-known point about muscles is that their variant force is determined by their length. A muscle actually creates its maximal force at an optimal length. That is why keeping your muscles at their optimal length is not just important for flexibility purposes, but also for optimal force and performance with the most efficiency and least chance of injury.

There are a series of lower body stretches that can be performed, including quad, hip flexor, hamstring, calf, piriformis, and ITB (iliotibial band) stretches. The upper body is less significant in terms of maintaining optimal length for one very important reason: we do not walk on our hands.

LOWER BODY STRETCHES

➤ Quad Stretch

Stretches the quads

Means of resistance: none

Lie on a surface with the leg to be stretched hanging off the side and the other leg on the surface with the knee bent and the foot on the surface. Next, place a towel around the ankle of the leg to be stretched in order to give you something to hold on to. Grab the towel and slowly begin to bend the knee toward the butt until a stretch is felt in the front of your thigh. Once you feel the stretch, hold it for 20 seconds and return to the start position. Make sure that your back does not arch while performing the stretch. This is a very stable position for stretching the quad and most people should be able to do this (versus the commonly suggested quad stretch of standing up and pulling the heel toward the butt).

Fig. 2-1. Quad stretch

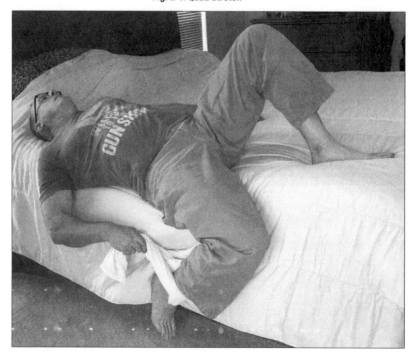

➤ Hip Flexor Stretch

Stretches the hip flexors

Means of resistance: none

Kneel down on one knee next to an object that will help you balance when performing this exercise, such as a chair or couch. The leg you are kneeling on is the one with the hip flexor that will be stretched. Slowly move the opposite leg in front of you with your other foot on the floor and the knee bent. Begin to move the pelvis forward with your torso upright so you start to move closer to the front foot. You will begin to feel a stretch at the upper thigh region of the leg you are kneeling on. Once a comfortable stretch is felt, hold it for 20 seconds.

Fig. 2-2. Hip flexor stretch

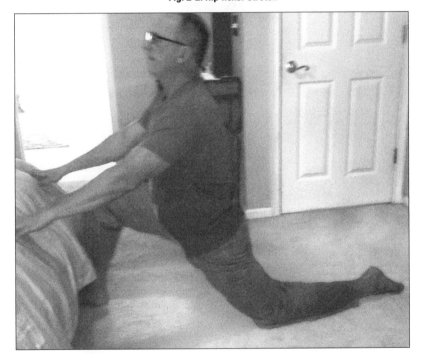

➤ **Hamstring Stretch**

Stretches the hamstrings

Means of resistance: none

Sitting on a surface with the leg to be stretched pointing in front of you and the other leg hanging off the side, place your hands on the thigh of the leg to be stretched. Make sure your back stays in a straight position and you don't hunch. Start to move your chest toward the leg out in front of you, keeping the knee unlocked and the toes pointing forward, away from your face. Continue to move the chest toward the leg until you feel a stretch at the back of the thigh. Once you feel the stretch, hold it for 20 seconds and return to the start position. You may not go too far before feeling the tightness at the back of the thigh. That's okay; you will improve over time.

Fig. 2-3. Hamstring stretch

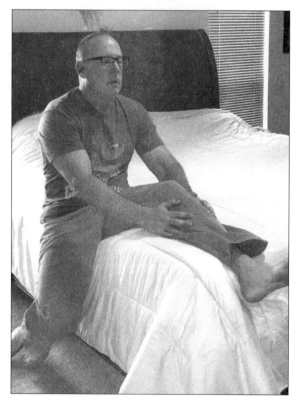

➤ Calf Stretch

Stretches the calf

Means of resistance: none

Stand in front of a wall. With your arms straight, place your hands on the wall. Keeping your feet hip width apart, bend one knee and step slightly back with your other foot. The calf of the back leg will be stretched. Make sure the whole foot stays on the floor during the stretch. Keeping the knee of the front leg bent, move your torso forward so more of your body weight is on the front leg. Continue moving forward until you feel a stretch in the back calf. Once you feel the stretch, hold it for 20 seconds and return to the start position.

Fig. 2-4. Calf stretch

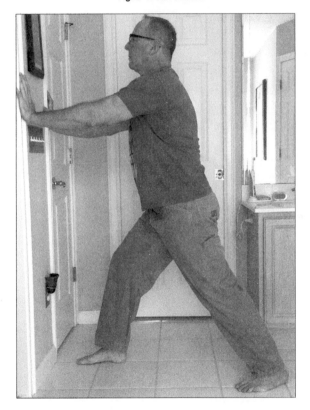

➤ **Piriformis Stretch**

Stretches the piriformis

Means of resistance: none

Sitting in a chair with your back supported, place the ankle of the leg to be stretched on the bent knee of the opposite leg. If the ankle cannot be placed on the knee, just place it as high up on the shin as possible. Then with both hands, grab the knee of the leg to be stretched. Pull the knee toward the opposite shoulder until a stretch is felt in the butt. Once you feel the stretch, hold it for 20 seconds and then return to the start position. This stretch can be used to diminish sciatic symptoms for short-term relief.

Fig. 2-5. Piriformis stretch

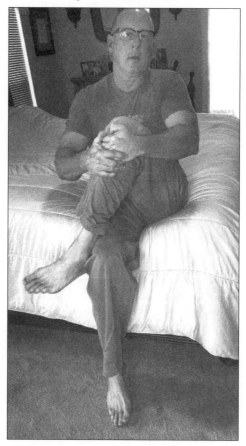

➤ ITB Stretch

Stretches the ITB

Means of resistance: none

Start by sitting in a chair with both feet on the floor. Place the ankle of the leg you are trying to stretch on the opposite knee. Put both hands on the knee of the leg you are trying to stretch and slowly press the knee down toward the floor, feeling a stretch at the outer thigh anywhere from the hip to the knee. Once a light stretch is felt, hold the position for 20 seconds. Then return to the start position. Your ITB may be too tight to be able to put the ankle on the opposite knee. If this is the case, start by placing the ankle halfway up the shin and holding it there with one hand while pressing down on the knee. This can be progressed until the ankle can finally be placed on the opposite knee to perform the stretch.

Fig. 2-6. ITB stretch

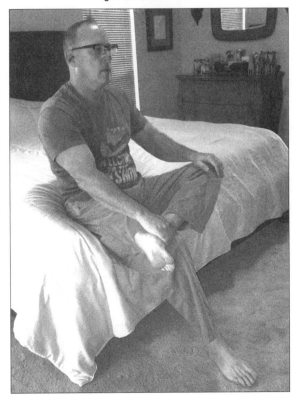

The fact that we walk on our legs means that the muscles of the legs are used throughout the course of the day at a much higher intensity, which is why they are more susceptible to straining and losing their optimal length. Probably the most significant upper body muscles that need to be stretched are the pecs, or chest muscles. The most common reason for upper back or neck pain and even migraine headaches is a muscle imbalance that develops between the pecs, front shoulder, and bicep versus the muscle between the shoulder blades, posterior shoulder, and tricep. This imbalance can create an improper posture known as "forward head and shoulder posture." As the shoulders are drawn forward, the shoulder blades themselves move away from the spine. Any muscle that attaches from the spine to the shoulder blade becomes overstretched and loses its ability to create force or perform a task. A muscle like the levator scapulae, which is responsible for supporting the head, can strain and emit pain at the neck and upper trapezius (trap) region and can even lead to headaches. Muscles like the middle trapezius (mid-trap) and rhomboids can strain and emit pain between the shoulder blades.

Fig. 2-7. Neck and shoulder muscles

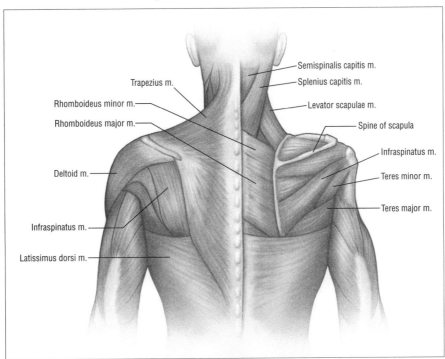

Trapezius m.

Rhomboideus minor m.

Rhomboideus major m.

Deltoid m.

Infraspinatus m.

Latissimus dorsi m.

Semispinalis capitis m.

Splenius capitis m.

Levator scapulae m.

Spine of scapula

Infraspinatus m.

Teres minor m.

Teres major m.

Fig. 2-8. Proper posture

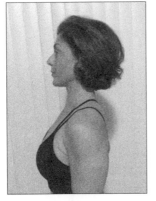

Fig. 2-9. Improper forward posture

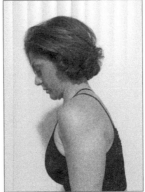

All of this is exaggerated the more the pecs are shortened. So if you are feeling increased pain at the neck, upper trap region, or between the shoulder blades, a good pec stretch might be the answer in the short term to decrease this pain.

➤ **Pec Stretch**

Stretches the pecs

Means of resistance: none

Stand in a doorway with your elbows at shoulder height. For those with long enough arms, the elbows will be sitting on the doorframe. If you have shorter arms, the elbows might be just inside the doorframe. With your feet centered in the doorway, begin to lean forward, keeping the torso upright. Your chest will begin to move slightly in front of the line of the shoulders, creating a pulling sensation at the front of the shoulders where the pecs attach to the shoulders. Move forward enough to create a light stretch. Hold this position for 20 seconds. Then return to the start position and repeat.

Fig. 2-10. Pec stretch

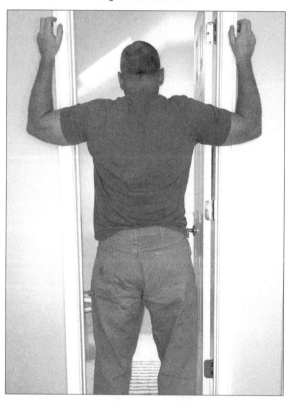

GETTING OUT OF BED

For many of you, getting out of bed may be the hardest thing you do in the entire day. The pain of moving from lying down to sitting up is devastating. Going from sitting at the end of the bed to standing can be just as hard. Trying to get to an upright standing position may seem to take herculean strength, effort, and a tremendous amount of pain. Many of you have been told this is because of the aging process or a herniated disc, stenosis, pinched nerve, or arthritis. Let me now introduce you to part of your body that you may not have known was responsible for this pain all along: the hip flexors.

The hip flexors are a group of muscles that attach from both the lumbar spine and the pelvis to the hip joint. The portions of the muscle group responsible for making standing upright so difficult are the psoas major and minor. These muscles attach from the lumbar spine and run on a diagonal through the abdominal cavity and end at the inner portion of the hip joint. They are called hip flexors because if you perceive the torso as the stable side of the muscle and the thigh connection as the moving side, the muscle brings the knee toward the chest. If you look at it from the reverse, with the leg as the stable side and the torso as the moving side, you would be bending forward, bringing the torso toward the ground. If the action of the hip flexors is to move the torso toward the ground, this means that the muscle shortens as this happens. That means that if you were to start to raise the torso toward moving upright again, this would cause the muscle to lengthen or stretch. So if the muscle were excessively shortened during the night, when you try to either sit up or stand up, the hip flexors would have a difficult time lengthening to allow the torso to move away from the thighs.

Fig. 2-11. Hip flexors

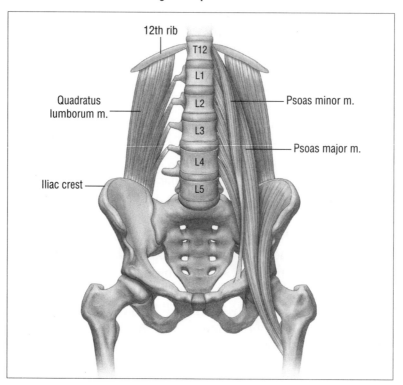

12th rib

T12

L1

Quadratus
lumborum m.

L2 — Psoas minor m.

L3

Psoas major m.

L4

Iliac crest

L5

A person with very shortened hip flexors oftentimes is a side sleeper who sleeps in a fetal position. This is where the hip flexors are allowed to be at their shortest. The downside of this is that when trying to go to a sitting position or, even worse, an upright standing position, the process of lengthening the muscles can create severe pain at the attachment to the lumbar spine. If this sounds like you and getting out of bed seems like an insurmountable challenge, let's try to take some of the difficulty out of it by addressing the cause.

Lengthening out the hip flexors should allow them to be flexible enough to enable you to go from lying to sitting to standing without pulling excessively on the lumbar spine. Remember that this is just a short-term mechanism designed to help you get through this aspect of the day. The long-term resolution of this problem will occur through the strengthening of the gluteus maximus muscles and the hamstrings. The gluteus maximus is the muscle found in the gluteal region, and the hamstrings are the posterior thigh muscles. These are the muscles that oppose the hip flexors and, when strengthened appropriately, will prevent the hip flexors from shortening again. The exercises to be performed are the hamstring curl, hip extension, and straight leg deadlifts. You will soon be able to hop out of bed with excitement and delight to see what the day will bring.

➤ Hamstring Curl: *Reverse Kick*

Strengthens the hamstrings

Means of resistance: machine or resistance band

In a seated position, place the resistance at the back of the ankle. Make sure you are supported in the seat (if you are using a machine, your lower back should be against the seat back; if you are using a resistance band/tube, position your butt about halfway to the front of the chair while you lean back with your shoulders supported by the chair back). Point your leg straight out with the knee unlocked. Bend the knee until it reaches 90 degrees. Then return to the start position. To isolate the hamstrings better, point the toes of the exercising leg toward your face as the exercise is being performed. In the case of using a seated hamstring curl machine, make sure the pivot point of the machine is aligned with the knee joint. If using a resistance band/tube, there may be a tendency for the knee to rise as the knee is bent. This is because the hamstrings are weak and the body is trying to compensate by using the hip flexors. To prevent this from occurring, place the hand on the same side of the body as the exercising leg on your knee as the exercise is performed. Prevent the knee from rising so that the foot just passes over the floor as the knee reaches 90 degrees of bend.

Fig. 2-12a. Start of hamstring curl

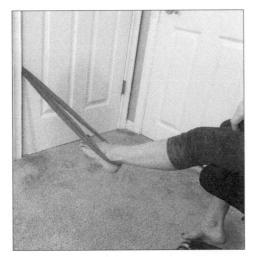

Fig. 2-12b. End of hamstring curl

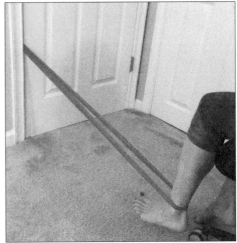

➤ **Hip Extension:** *Kick Back*

Strengthens the gluteus maximus

Means of resistance: machine or resistance band

In a standing position, place the resistance between the door and frame at knee height and then behind your knee. Place the standing leg behind you so it causes you to weight bear against the door and wall with both hands. This will make you feel like you are leaning against the door and wall more than standing on one leg, which will help you to kick behind you without trying to move your body with the leg that is moving. Take the leg that is exercising and bend the knee to 90 degrees. Point the toes forward so the heel leads the foot moving backward. The knee of the working leg should be at least six inches in front of the standing leg's knee at the start. Start to kick behind you until the thigh of the moving leg is in line with the thigh of the standing leg. Then return to the start position. The key to this exercise is for there to be no lateral motion of the body or bending forward and back of the torso. The only thing moving should be the working thigh. Try to keep your back rounded or at least flat so you do not arch the lower back during any part of the exercise.

Fig. 2-13a. Start of hip extension

Fig. 2-13b. End of hip extension

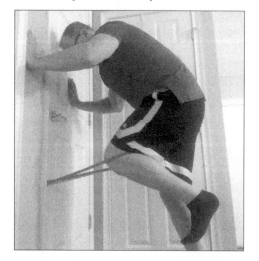

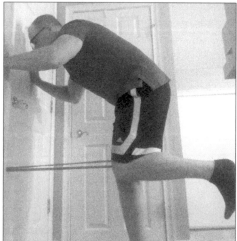

➤ Straight Leg Deadlifts: *Run the Hands down the Thighs*

Strengthens the gluteus maximus and hamstrings

Means of resistance: dumbbells or resistance band

Start with your feet a little more than shoulder width apart and your toes pointing slightly out. You should be standing straight with your knees unlocked and your butt pushed back slightly. Hold the resistance in front of your thighs. Bend from the hips, keeping your back straight while looking out in front of you, and begin to lower the resistance down your legs. Make sure your knees don't bend and the motion is coming from your hips. As you move down, you should feel your weight shift to your heels. When you begin to feel tightness at the back of your thighs, slowly straighten back up to the start position. There is no specific point to reach down on the leg. Reach down until you feel tightness at the back of your thighs. Make sure your back remains straight, not rounded. If it's rounded, you can strain your back and you will also go down farther than you could with a straight back. As you go down, you will feel your weight shift back onto your heels. Make sure that the resistance is held tight to your thighs throughout the whole exercise.

Fig. 2-14a. Start of straight leg deadlifts

Fig. 2-14b. End of straight leg deadlifts

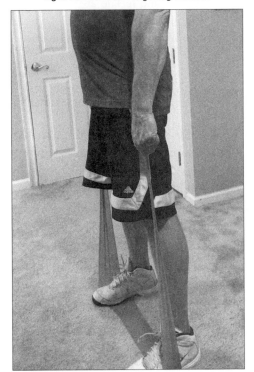
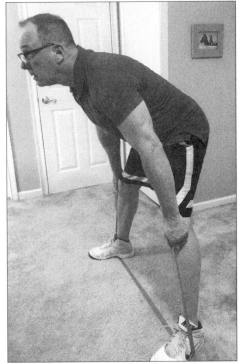

➤ **Hip Flexor Stretch**

See p. 206 for instructions.

Fig. 2-15. Hip flexor stretch

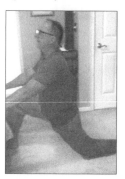

For those who wake up with back pain or would like to stretch before getting out of bed, lie on the side of the bed so that one leg can hang off the bed while the other leg is bent and the foot placed on the bed. Be careful to slowly lower the leg off the side of the bed, ensuring that the other leg is bent and the foot on the bed before doing so. For many of you, this will create a severe stretching feeling at the upper front thigh of the leg that is hanging, stretching the hip flexors. Hold this stretch for 20 seconds, then bring the leg back up on the bed and wait about 30 seconds before performing the stretch again. Do this stretch on both sides of the bed for both legs.

MORNING ROUTINES

Morning routines can oftentimes be chaotic. For many, it is a race against time to get ready and begin the day. Activities are often performed without thought or perfect mechanics. This can lead muscles to overwork and strain, ultimately eliciting pain. A cultural precept has developed that leads people to the wrong conclusion about how to respond when they have pain while performing an activity. Are you familiar with the old joke, "'Doc, it hurts when I do this,' and the doctor replies, 'Then don't do it!'"? The premise here is that if something creates pain, then you shouldn't do that activity. This is a very dangerous, not to mention impractical, mind-set to develop. What must be understood is that activities and tasks are performed by many muscles working together.

What if the activity in question is something a person really likes to do or has to do? Asking the person to not do that activity can limit their quality of life or can even limit their ability to make a living. What I would propose instead is a mind-set that says if there is pain when performing a task, you should identify which muscle is strained or imbalanced and correct the deficit. Once the deficit is resolved, the activity can be performed with ease and without eliciting pain. This is the attitude that will ultimately enable people to be able to live their lives performing whatever activities they choose.

TEETH BRUSHING AND HAIR DRYING

I have treated many a patient who felt that brushing their teeth was one of the most difficult activities to perform in the morning because of significant back pain. What must be understood is that there has to have been a predisposition for some muscles to strain for this simple act to trigger a severe level of back pain. The muscles most associated with centralized lower back pain are the hip flexors. This muscle group is primarily made up of the psoas major and minor, which actually attaches to the lumbar spine and runs down through the abdominal cavity to the hip joints. This muscle group has a natural tendency to be stronger than its opposing muscle group, the gluteus maximus (muscle in the buttocks region). If this imbalance becomes too great, the hip flexors will have a tendency to shorten. In shortening, the muscles become susceptible to spasm.

When you are brushing your teeth, you typically lean forward so that the toothpaste lands in the sink rather than the floor. This is a mildly hip-flexed position. It can be sustained for a couple of minutes, depending on how long you brush your teeth. If sustained for a long enough period to where the hip flexors shorten enough to go into spasm, it can create a massive level of pain at the lower back where the hip flexor muscles attach to the lumbar spine. This could be enough pain to prevent you from supporting your torso and force you to sit down or even end up on the floor.

The remedy for this problem is to stretch the hip flexors and strengthen the gluteus maximus and hamstrings. By stretching the hip flexors, you will be lengthening them and strengthening the hamstrings and gluteus maximus, which will let you sustain the length of the hip flexors. This will prevent straining, spasm, or lower back pain.

Blow-drying your hair can create the same sort of pain, particularly if you're someone who tends to lean into the mirror to see what you're doing. This forces your torso into a hip-flexed position, again leading to shortening of the hip flexors and the possibility of lower back pain. The other elements involved in this activity are the support of the blow-dryer and your arm above shoulder height. This might not seem like a major load to support, but to do so for the time it takes to blow-dry one's hair can actually be pretty stressful to the shoulder and shoulder blade muscles.

The shoulder joint is really the arm attaching into the end of the shoulder blade. The shoulder blade sits on the rib cage, but it is not attached by any ligaments or joint capsule. It is held together by muscles, so the strength of the shoulder joint is only as strong as the support of the shoulder blade against the rib cage. In order to perform an action like blow-drying your hair, I would suggest strengthening the key muscles of the shoulder and shoulder blade, including the posterior deltoids, the rotator cuff, the lower trapezius (trap), the rhomboids/mid-traps, and the triceps. To strengthen the posterior deltoid, perform the posterior deltoid exercise. To strengthen the rotator cuff, perform external rotation. To strengthen the lower trapezius muscle, perform the lower trap exercise. To strengthen the rhomboids/mid-traps, perform lat pulldowns with neutral bar. To strengthen the triceps, perform tricep extension.

➤ **Posterior Deltoids:** *Gorilla Arms*

Strengthens the posterior deltoids

Means of resistance: dumbbells or resistance band

Stand with your feet more than shoulder width apart, knees slightly bent, and your butt pushed behind you so that you are bending forward slightly. Your weight should be mostly on your heels. Hold the resistance in front of your thighs with your palms facing in and your elbows unlocked (if using resistance bands or tubes, your arms will be at the side of your legs, touching them to start the exercise). Begin to move the resistance out to your side from the shoulders like a pendulum. Go out until you feel your shoulder blades start to move inward (about 60 degrees), and then return to the beginning position.

Fig. 2-16a. Beginning of posterior deltoid exercise

Fig. 2-16b. End of posterior deltoid exercise

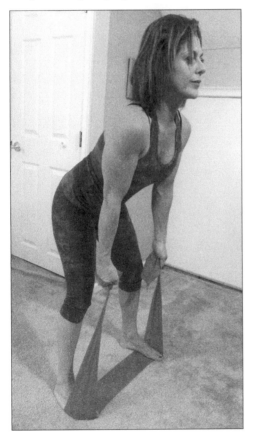

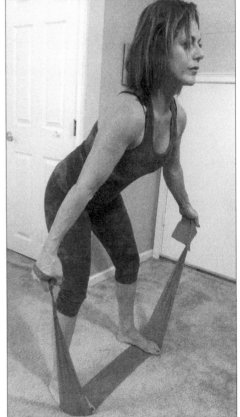

➤ External Rotation: *Reverse Hammering*

Strengthens the rotator cuff

Means of resistance: dumbbell or resistance band

With the elbow supported at the end of a surface or on a doorknob so that the elbow is just below shoulder height, maintain the elbow at a 90-degree angle through the whole motion. The elbow of the arm performing the exercise should be in a line with both shoulders (if the elbow is in front of this line, the rotator cuff will have difficulty performing the exercise). The start position is with the forearm facing about 20 degrees below parallel to the ground. The resistance is pulled upward until the forearm is facing about 20 degrees above parallel. Then return to the start position. Keep the range of motion as described. Excessive motion can lead to the rotator cuff straining.

Fig. 2-17a. Beginning of external rotation   **Fig. 2-17b. End of external rotation**

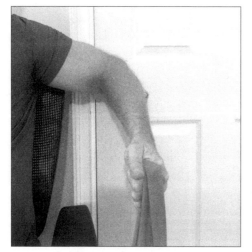
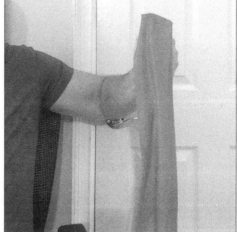

➤ **Lower Trap:** *Paint the Wall*

Strengthens the lower trapezius muscle

Means of resistance: dumbbell or resistance band

This exercise is critical to achieving complete functional capacity of the shoulder. Sit in a sturdy chair and lean back slightly with your butt halfway toward the front of the chair and your back resting against the seat back. If you have difficulty supporting your head while performing this exercise, place the chair against a wall so you can support your head against the wall to prevent the resistance from pulling you forward. Start with your arm halfway between pointing straight forward and pointing straight to the side, with your hand at eye level and your elbow just unlocked. Your palm will be facing in as you grab the resistance. Begin to raise the resistance until the upper arm is in line with the cheek. Then return to the start position at shoulder height. I like to describe this as moving from eye to cheek. Keep in mind that the muscle creating the motion that appears to be occurring at the shoulder is actually at the lower thoracic region and pulling your shoulder blade down your back, which ultimately causes the arm to rise at the shoulder. Try to imagine your shoulder blade being pulled down your back or have somebody put their hand on your shoulder blade so you can feel your shoulder blade moving down the back.

Fig. 2-18a. Beginning of lower trap exercise

Fig. 2-18b. End of lower trap exercise

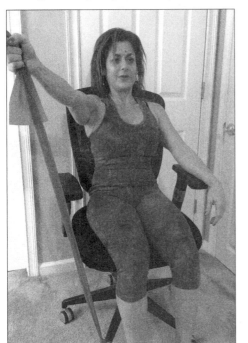
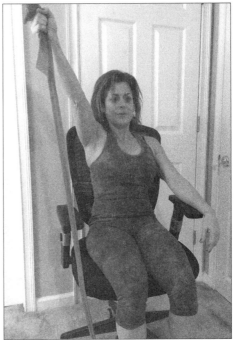

➤ **Lat Pulldown with Neutral Bar:** *Pull Down from Shelf*

Strengthens the interscapular muscles: mid-traps and rhomboids

Means of resistance: Neutral bar or elastic band

Leaning back with an angle at the hip of about 30 degrees (if sitting in a chair, have your butt halfway to the front of the chair while your shoulders are leaning against the seat back), reach up for the bar or elastic band so that the start position begins with your arms nearly straight and your elbows just unlocked. Your feet should be flat on the floor in front of you. Pull the mechanism down, keeping your elbows at shoulder height until your elbows reach just behind the line of your shoulders. The forearms should be maintained in a continuous line with the resistance. Then return to the start position. Don't let your elbows fall during the motion. This will cause you to work a different muscle than the muscles between the shoulder blades.

Fig. 2-19a. Beginning of lat pulldown   **Fig. 2-19b. End of lat pulldown**

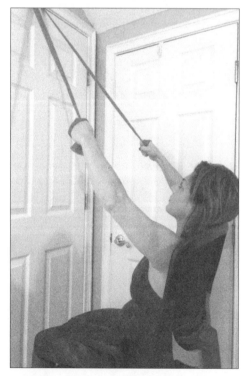
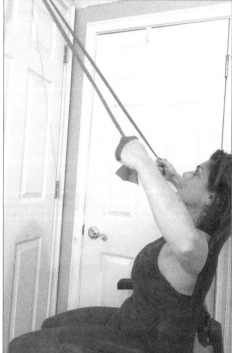

➤ Tricep Extensions: *Casting a Fishing Rod*

Strengthens the triceps, single and both arms

Means of resistance: dumbbells, EZ curl bar, or resistance band

This exercise is the most effective way to strengthen the triceps because it puts the long head of the triceps in the optimal position. The long head of the triceps is the only part of the triceps muscle that passes the shoulder joint. Therefore, it is the only part of the muscle that can affect the position of the arm bone in the shoulder joint. This exercise can be performed with one arm or both, depending on whether your pain is associated with one side or requires both arms to be strengthened to resolve it. To perform the exercise, lie on your back with your feet supported on the floor. Start with your arms pointing straight up over the shoulders, with your elbows just unlocked. Keeping your upper arms in place, begin to bend your elbows, lowering your forearms so your hands and resistance are moving toward your forehead. Once your elbows reach 90 degrees, return to the start position. Make sure not to lock the elbows at the top of the motion. (If performing the exercise with a resistance band or tube, sit in a chair with your back to the door and your back supported by the back rest with your feet on the floor in front of you. The resistance band should be set between the door and frame just above head height, and your elbow should be at shoulder height. Grab the resistance band with your elbow at a 90-degree angle and with the palm facing inward, straighten your elbow, keeping the upper arm level until just before the elbow locks. Then return to the start position.)

Fig. 2-20a. Beginning of tricep extensions

Fig. 2-20b. End of tricep extensions

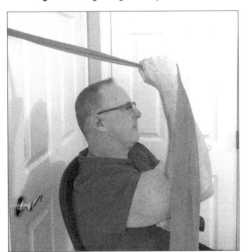
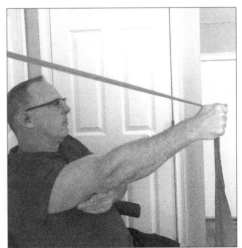

GETTING DRESSED

Getting dressed can present a slew of obstacles for those who are not appropriately conditioned. Dressing without the fear of pain or injury requires full range of joint motion and the flexibility and strength of the relevant muscles.

Putting on your pants can be complicated if you have muscle flexibility deficits that prevent you from stretching enough to reach your feet and place them through the legs of the pants. You might need to put the pants on the floor, step into the legs, and find a way to reach down to pick up the pants or even use some assistive device to reach them. In such cases, there is one primary reason the limitation might occur: an imbalance between the quadricep muscles and hamstrings.

Fig. 2-21. Quads

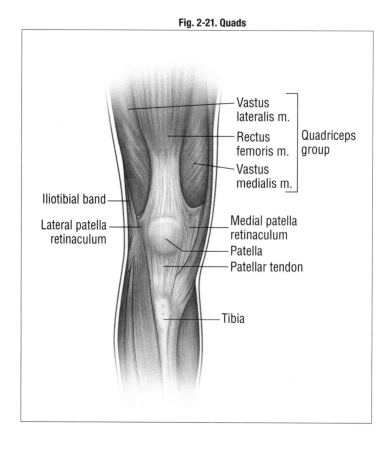

Fig. 2-22. Hamstrings

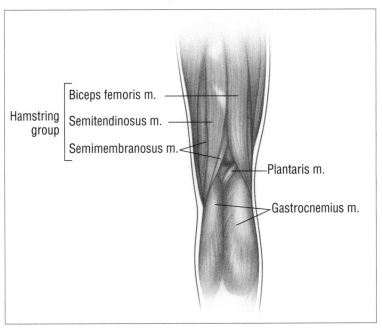

If you are having problems leaning forward to dress, you most likely have difficulty bending forward at the hip. This might cause a severe arching of the lower back wherein the curve cannot reverse to allow for the complete range of motion that should be available at the lower back. The normal motion of the lower back should be in a mild arch at regular stance, but when bending forward the curve of the lower back should be able to reverse to allow the lower back to bend optimally. The limitation in this ability to reverse the curve when bending forward is most often associated with a muscle imbalance between the quads (front thigh) and hamstrings (posterior thigh). A natural imbalance usually exists because you use your quads for most weight-bearing activities, such as sitting, standing, negotiating stairs, or walking. But if this imbalance becomes too great, then the quads will have a tendency to shorten substantially. Since the quads are attached to the front of the pelvis, it will pull the front of the pelvis down, causing the back of the pelvis to rise. This leads to excessive arching of the lower back. In this altered posture, the lower back muscles (which attach from the bottom of the rib cage to the top of pelvis) will shorten severely. When you want to bend forward, as you would when putting pants on, the shortened lower back muscles will no longer stretch to their optimal length, which prevents the lower back going from an arched position to a hunched position. This is what stops you from being able to bend forward enough to reach your feet.

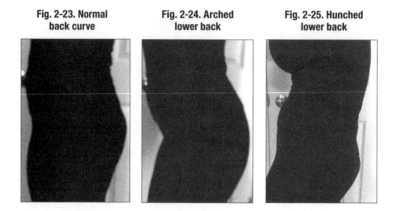

Fig. 2-23. Normal back curve **Fig. 2-24. Arched lower back** **Fig. 2-25. Hunched lower back**

To resolve this problem, stretch the quads and strengthen the hamstrings and gluteus maximus muscles. These are the muscles that oppose the quads and will sustain their length. Once the quads are maintained at their optimal length, the arch of the lower back will no longer be able to increase and the lower back muscles will sustain their optimal length for full range of motion. The exercises to perform include a quad stretch, hamstring curl, and hip extension.

➤ **Quad Stretch**

See p. 208 for instructions.

Fig. 2-26. Quad stretch

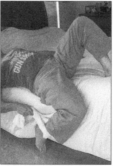

➤ **Hamstring Curl:** *Reverse Kick*

See p. 196 for instructions.

See p. 196 for instructions.

Fig. 2-27a. Beginning of hamstring curl

Fig. 2-27b. End of hamstring curl

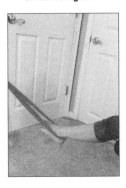 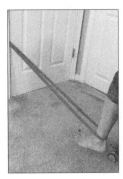

➤ **Hip Extension:** *Kick Back*

See p. 198 for instructions.

Fig. 2-28a. Beginning of hip extension

Fig. 2-28b. End of hip extension

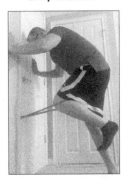 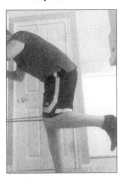

One point about this issue I would like to make is that there is a pervasive notion that limited lower back range of motion is due to tight hamstrings (the back of the thigh muscle). However, more than 90 percent of people I have treated with this problem have ultimately turned out to have tight quads (front thigh muscles), whereas the hamstrings were actually hyperflexible.

**Fig. 2-29a. Proper
flexibility of hamstrings**

**Fig. 2-29b. Hyper
flexibility of hamstrings**

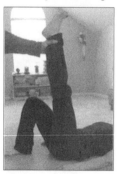
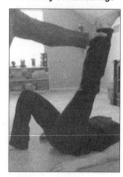

The simplest way to determine this is to check the flexibility of the quads and hamstrings by performing the stretching techniques for each and looking at the lower back to see if it is more arched or flattened with a limited arch. If the back is excessively arched, the quads are too tight. If it is flattened, then the hamstrings are too tight. Most people upon examination will find they are excessively arched.

**Fig. 2-30. Quad
flexibility test**

Fig. 2-31. Arched back

**Fig. 2-32. Hamstring
flexibility test**

**Fig. 2-33. Flattened
lower back**

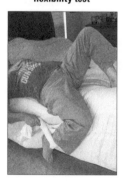
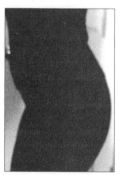
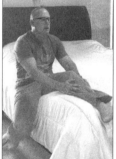
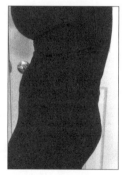

Even if you complete all of the recommended exercises and develop the ability to reach your feet and place them through the pant legs, there is one other possible obstacle to completing this task: standing up and balancing yourself to lift the pants up and secure them. Balance, for many, can be a problem because balance is determined by the ear and brain's understanding of where you are in space. So if you can sit without any support of the hands or sides of a chair and you are stable, the neurological part of balance must be working properly. But if you then find it difficult to remain stable while standing, the muscles of the legs are weak.

The muscles most associated with balance are the gluteus medius muscles. These muscles sit to the side of the pelvis, just above the hip joint, and are responsible for keeping the pelvis level, especially when single-leg standing—such as when you put on your pants one foot at a time. If this muscle is weak, then you will feel like you will fall toward the opposite side of the body you are balancing on. This is the main reason people do not have stable balance.

The remedy to this issue is strengthening the gluteus medius muscles. To achieve this, perform the hip abduction exercise.

➤ Hip Abduction: *Side Step*

Strengthens the gluteus medius

Means of resistance: cable machine or resistance band

Hip abductions can be performed either lying on your side or standing. To do this exercise correctly, make sure you do not move your leg too far outward. There may be a false sense that more range of motion is better, but in this case, too much range of motion means you are using the lower back muscle to create the motion, not the gluteus medius (hip muscle). The gluteus medius muscle can only move the leg out to the point where the outer portion of the ankle is in line with the outer portion of the hip joint. Any outward motion beyond that is created by the lower back muscle. To do the exercise, lie on your side with the knee of the bottom leg bent and the top leg straight. The top leg should run in a continuous line from the torso. If the leg is angled in front of the torso, you are using a different muscle than the gluteus medius. Start to raise the top leg off the supporting leg until your leg is parallel with the floor. Try to turn the leg in slightly so the heel is the first part of the foot that is moving. This puts the gluteus medius in the optimal position to raise the leg. Once your leg reaches parallel to the floor, begin to lower back onto the supporting leg.

If performing this exercise standing, start with the feet together with the resistance connected to the ankle. Turn the working leg's foot in slightly so the heel is the first part of the foot to move to the side. Step out to the side until the outer portion of the ankle meets the outer portion of the hip. Place this foot on the floor and weight bear fully on it, taking the load off the other foot. Then return the foot back to the start position next to the other foot. Make sure that when you move the working foot out to the side that you are pushing yourself over with the foot you are weight bearing on. Focus your attention on moving the exercised leg over. You may be very weak and feel that you require arm support to perform the exercise correctly. You can place a chair in front of you with the chair back facing you so that you can hold on to it with your hands. The key is not to use this to support yourself beyond what is required.

Fig. 2-34a. Beginning of hip abduction

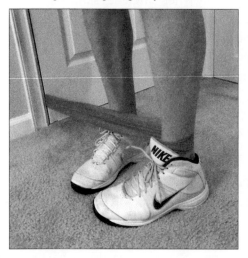

Fig. 2-34b. End of hip abduction

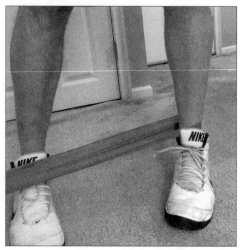

Fig. 2-34c. Beginning of hip abduction

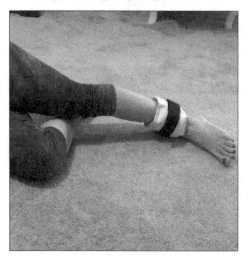

Fig. 2-34d. End of hip abduction

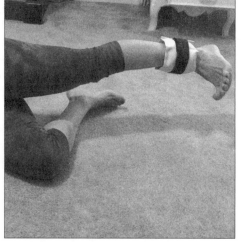

Fig. 2-34e. Side view of hip abduction

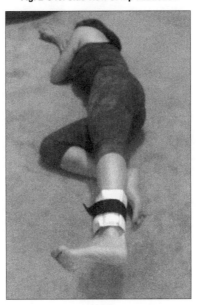

Now let's talk about putting your socks and shoes on. This is a real struggle for many people because they can't put one ankle on the opposing knee in order to place the sock and shoe on one foot. The person is often told they have arthritis of the hip and there is nothing that can be done about this circumstance, so they start to use assistive devices or are simply left to struggle. I have known people who stopped purchasing lace-up shoes and went to only wearing slip-ons. These might seem like somewhat mundane decisions, but why should we have to make them? Why must we give up hope of ever achieving something that doesn't need to be difficult?

For most people who have difficulty placing one ankle on the opposite knee when sitting, there is tightness at the lateral aspect of the thigh being raised. As the foot is raised, the knee will not bend to the side and will continue to rise with the foot. Eventually there is no way to raise the foot higher, so it can't reach the opposite knee. The limitation of the knee moving to the side is due to a tight ITB band (iliotibial band). This is a thick connective band that runs from the hip region down the side of the lateral aspect of the thigh to the knee.

Fig. 2-35. ITB (side of thigh)

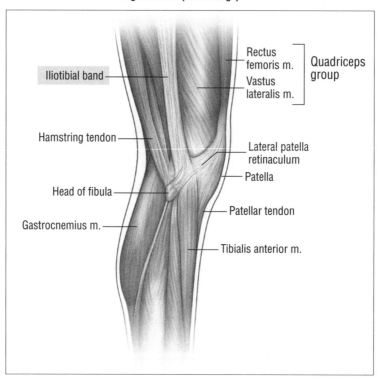

When this is shortened, it will not allow rotation at the hip to occur, which is required for the knee to fall to the side when placing the foot on the opposing knee. The ITB will strain and shorten when the gluteus medius muscle (the muscle that supports you when single-leg standing) strains. This muscle sits just above the hip joint and works with the ITB band along with the small muscle that sits at the top of the band, called the tensor fascia lata. If the gluteus medius muscle strains, the ITB band and tensor fascia lata will overwork, strain, and shorten. Once the ITB has shortened, it becomes difficult for the knee to fall to the side, and therefore difficult to place the foot on the opposite knee.

To resolve this issue, stretch the ITB and strengthen the gluteus medius and quads to prevent the ITB and tensor fascia lata from straining and shortening. The exercises to be performed include the ITB stretch, hip abduction, and knee extension.

➤ **ITB Stretch**

See p. 207 for instructions.

Fig. 2-36. ITB stretch

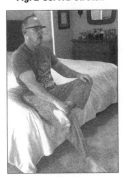

➤ **Hip Abduction:** *Side Step*

See p. 196 for instructions.

Fig. 2-37a. Beginning of hip abduction exercise

Fig. 2-37b. End of hip abduction exercise

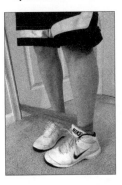

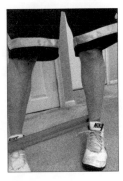

Fig. 2-37c. Beginning of hip abduction exercise

Fig. 2-37d. End of hip abduction exercise

Fig. 2-37e. Side view of hip abduction exercise

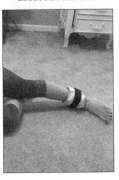

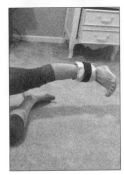

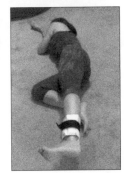

➤ **Knee Extension:** *Seated Kick*

Strengthens the quads

Means of resistance: machine or resistance band

In a seated position, place the resistance around the front of the ankle. Make sure the foot of the opposite leg is on the floor and you are supported in a seat. Begin with the knee bent to 90 degrees; then straighten the knee until it is almost locked. Then return the leg to the start position. Make sure the thigh of the leg that is being exercised remains on the seat and does not rise with the lower leg. If performing with a resistance band/tube, place the resistance under the front leg of the chair next to the working leg. Make sure you make a small loop with the band/tube because you are going to want resistance immediately upon performing the motion of the exercise.

Fig. 2-38a. Beginning of knee extension

Fig. 2-38b. End of knee extension

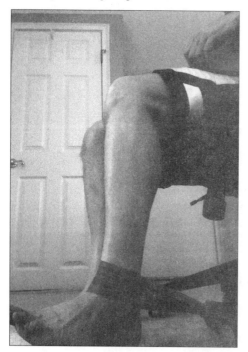

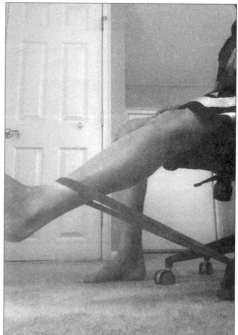

Putting on a belt or a bra can become troublesome if the rotator cuff strains and shortens. For these two tasks, the key is being able to place your hand behind the back to either secure the bra or to place the belt through the back loops of the pants. The rotator cuff is unique in that it is responsible for keeping the arm bone in the shoulder joint through 360 degrees of motion. So it must be flexible enough to go through that range of motion, but strong enough to create support. This makes it susceptible to straining. If strained enough, the muscles will shorten, making it more difficult to place your hand behind your back.

To resolve this issue, you must first perform internal rotation of the shoulder to lengthen the rotator cuff. Once it feels as easy to place the hand behind the back on the affected side as it does on the unaffected side, you can switch to performing external rotation to strengthen the rotator cuff to prevent it from straining and shortening again. Since shoulder function is the product of a group of muscles working together, strengthen the posterior deltoid, rhomboids/ mid-traps, lower trap, and triceps by performing the posterior deltoids, lat pull-down with neutral bar, lower trap, and tricep extension. Also continue the process of lengthening and strengthening the rotator cuff.

➤ Posterior Deltoids: *Gorilla Arms*

See p. 191 for instructions.

Fig. 2-39a. Beginning of posterior deltoids exercise	Fig. 2-39b. End of posterior deltoids exercise

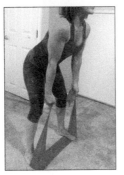
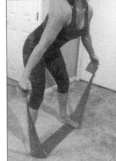

➤ **Lat Pulldown with Neutral Bar:** *Pull Down from Shelf*

See p. 190 for instructions.

Fig. 2-40a. Beginning of lat pulldown

Fig. 2-40b. End of lat pulldown

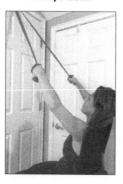 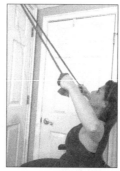

➤ **Lower Trap:** *Paint the Wall*

See p. 190 for instructions.

Fig. 2-41a. Beginning of lower trap exercise

Fig. 2-41b. End of lower trap exercise

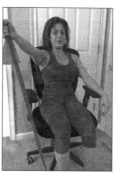 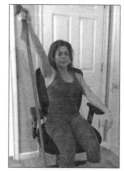

PROACTIVELY PLANNING YOUR DAY

When getting ready for your day, you try to think about what you will be doing and where you will be so that you can prepare for what lies ahead. If you are going to be driving a lot, you might gas up the car the day before since anxiety about racing to get gas on the way to other appointments can cause increased stress at the neck and lower back, which can lead to muscles tightening and straining. Find a quiet spot to stop and unwind, take a walk, or do some calisthenics. If you have to do a lot of traveling during the day, plan to wear more comfortable shoes like sneakers and bring a change of shoes for the rest of the day. If at all possible, see if you can schedule time at a gym for a half hour to an hour to perform some exercises (this only has to be done two or three times a week). Not only can you get some valuable exercise time, but it is also a great way to break up the day and give your head a break from all your other responsibilities.

If you have to carry a lot with you for the day, try to disperse the items between both arms or use a backpack-style of bag to hold the items. When using a pocketbook or a bag with a single shoulder strap, you are placing more weight on one side of the body than the other, which can lead to straining for the muscles burdened with the excess load. If your job requires you to sit for many hours, try to create situations that allow you to incorporate some type of walking during the course of the day. Maybe park a little farther away from your destination so you need to walk a bit to get there. Take the stairs versus the elevator on occasion.

Muscles that are not used will weaken. You need to sustain the strength of your muscles by activating them during the course of the day. True, these additional steps will not build muscle or make them stronger—that comes with strength training, which I recommend everybody perform two to three times a week. But even with strength training, if the muscles are left continuously inactive throughout the day, they will have a tendency to weaken, leaving them susceptible to straining when called upon to do an activity or task.

OUT THE DOOR AND ON YOUR WAY

Hopefully the steps I have previously outlined will make you feel more energetic and less symptomatic as you start your day. If you are in pain in the morning, it will carry over to the rest of the day and make the day feel like it is a lot longer and more difficult. Try to address the issues you might be having in the morning so you can embark on the rest of the day rested, limber, and energetic. I have treated many people who describe one of their symptoms as being tired a lot during the day. Remember, if your muscles are not strong and balanced, they will be inefficient in how they produce force, making activities and tasks seem harder than they should be. Greater energy is needed because the muscles are not able to do as much as they would if they were at their optimal performance level. This could be the reason that you might feel tired by the afternoon or early evening. If you are having pain that makes you feel like you're dragging through the day, try to resolve the causes of your pain on a muscular level—you might find a whole lot of energy being released and newly available for you.

CHAPTER THREE

At Work

DO YOU SIT FOR A LIVING?

Since the advent of the computer, more and more people find themselves spending much of their day sitting for their jobs. Sitting for long periods of time is a detriment to maintaining strength and balance. This lack of muscle usage can also eventually result in pain. You can see the consequences of lack of muscle use in other situations such as when astronauts live on a space station for an extended period of time without gravity. Because they do not have to support their body weight or use their muscles, they inevitably lose muscle mass and experience atrophy. Another example is when a person has been ill for a while and bedridden. Due to the lack of use of the leg muscles, atrophy occurs and can be seen in the difficulty in performing weight-bearing activities.

While walking or performing weight-bearing activity is not going to resolve the cause of pain, it certainly can contribute to the possibility of muscles straining if they are not activated over the course of the day.

Although sitting requires little energy to perform and is sedentary by nature, it actually must be perceived as an *activity*. I consider any action where muscle length is altered to be an activity.

When you are standing or lying on your back, the thigh runs continuously in line with the torso. This means that the angle between the thigh and torso is 180 degrees. When you sit, the angle changes dramatically to 90 degrees, which allows the hip flexors to shorten severely. For most people, an insignificant muscle imbalance exists between the hip flexors and its opposing muscle group, the gluteus maximus muscle. With enough pulling from the gluteus maximus muscle, the hip flexors will not shorten significantly. Therefore, the hip flexors in this minimally shortened state will not develop extensive tension and lower back pain will not develop.

When standing or lying down, the normal position of the lower back is a mild arch. When sitting is attempted, this should be able to transition to a mild hunch. When flexibility in the lumbar region allows both the hip flexors and lower back muscles to stretch without creating pain, the hip flexors can be sustained at their proper length. However, if the hip flexors are significantly stronger than the gluteus maximus muscles, then they will shorten and pull excessively on their attachment to the lumbar spine. This force will present itself as the lower back being pulled into the stomach. Excessive arching of the lower back will then also be seen in standing. When sitting is attempted in this scenario, the lumber spine will not be able to go from mildly arched to mildly hunched. Tension will build in the hip flexors because they are being overly shortened. Eventually, pain will develop at the lumbar spine region and the person will feel that they can no longer sit or will have to constantly readjust their position.

As painful as sitting can be, the real difficulty can occur when a person tries to stand up. Standing up requires the angle between the torso and the thigh to go from 90 degrees to 180 degrees instantly. If the hip flexors are shortened, they will not be able to lengthen back as quickly as is needed. Severe pain will occur at the lumbar spine where the hip flexors are attached and pulling excessively. The person may feel like they need to support their torso weight with their hands on their thighs. They will then feel that they need to push their torsos to an upright position by running their hands up their thighs. At some point the tension should begin to diminish and standing upright should be able to be achieved. For some, however, this can actually cause the hip flexors to go into spasm, and the pain at the lumbar spine will be too great and force them to sit down.

The resolution to this entire dilemma is to keep your hip flexors lengthened by stretching them and strengthening the gluteus maximus muscles and hamstrings. The exercises to perform are hip flexor stretch, hip extension, hamstring curl, and straight leg deadlifts.

➤ Hip Flexor Stretch

See p. 206 for instructions.

Fig. 3-1. Hip flexor stretch

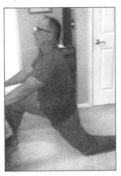

➤ Hip Extension: *Kick Back*

See p. 198 for instructions.

Fig. 3-2a. Beginning of hip extension

Fig. 3-2b. End of hip extension

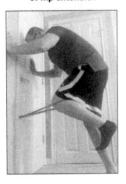 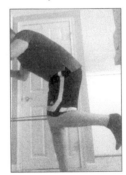

➤ **Hamstring Curl:** *Reverse Kick*

See p. 196 for instructions.

Fig. 3-3a. Beginning of hamstring curl

Fig. 3-3b. End of hamstring curl

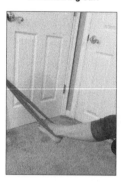
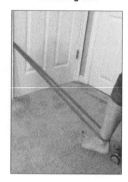

➤ **Straight Leg Deadlifts:** *Run the Hands down the Thighs*

See p. 204 for instructions.

Fig. 3-4a. Beginning of straight leg deadlifts

Fig. 3-4b. End of straight leg deadlifts

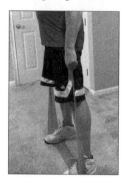
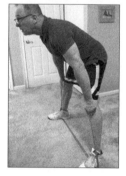

These exercises will give your spine the ability to go from a mildly arched position in standing to a mildly hunched position in sitting with no tension developing in the lower back region. Sitting will become a tolerable activity, allowing you to focus without the constant feeling of tension and pain at the lower back.

Because this issue is so widespread, and the average person has no idea why sitting leads to such significant lower back pain, a cottage industry has developed. The standing desk has become a craze in society under the assumption that because a person no longer has to sit, lower back pain can be avoided. Then, of course, there are those who promote sitting on a therapy ball with the idea that you will use your abdominal muscles more, thus supporting your lower back.

With regard to the standing desk, while you are no longer sitting and are avoiding the change in angle between the torso and thigh, you are still performing an activity that requires groups of muscles. All the muscles required for standing will then need to be isolated and strengthened. If not, you will eventually stand in an altered manner, causing different muscles to break down and creating pain in other areas.

As for sitting on a therapy ball, the ball is clearly an unstable surface. As a result, muscles required to create stability must be incorporated to develop the support that a solid chair would achieve. This means energy must be expended by these now supporting muscles. Muscles like the gluteus medius must become engaged, and the abdominal and lower back muscles must also engage. The quads and hamstrings must help to brace the body by creating force through the feet. The trouble with the unstable therapy ball is that your energy expenditure for simply sitting will rise dramatically, causing you to utilize energy at a much quicker speed and experience greater fatigue over the course of the day. If the argument is that you are performing a form of exercise during the day that helps to activate muscles that would otherwise remain inactive while sitting, it must be understood that this has nothing to do with reducing the chance of back pain and, in fact, will most likely increase it.

If the goal is to perform exercise during the course of the day to offset the lack of activity that comes with a sitting job, I would prefer that targeted strength training be performed with resistance bands either at your desk or in a break room and for you to combine this with taking walks or using stairs. With the Yass Method, targeted exercises are performed on a single plane—forward/back, side to side, or parallel to the ground—to isolate individual muscles. Therefore, the exercises are simple to perform.

Most of the exercises can be performed in a sitting position, and the majority of the standing exercises are performed with one foot on the floor with the support of the arms. Resistance can be developed through the use of resistance bands that can be attached to a desk, chair, or doorway, so no other equipment is needed. This type of exercise isolates all muscles, allowing strong and balanced muscles to be developed. The skeleton and muscles will be worked to maximize function and limit injury, preventing the development of pain.

HOW PHYSICAL IS YOUR WORK?

Activity does not resolve pain that is caused by muscle weakness or imbalance, but it does sustain the strength of the muscle once it is developed. So being active as part of your day is essential to sustaining strength and muscle balance.

For a person who sits for most of the workday, there is a high probability that their muscles are becoming weaker from lack of use. This won't affect that person during the workweek because the force requirements of the job are less than the force output of the muscles performing the job. But what happens when the person decides they want to garden over the weekend or clean their home or play a sport? Suddenly the force requirements of these activities are much greater than the force output of the muscles that have been weakened due to lack of use. This is a classic setup for these muscles to be strained and to create pain.

This is why I wholeheartedly endorse finding a half hour three to five times a week to do an isolated strength-training workout and to do some other physical activity like walking or climbing stairs when you have a job that requires sitting most of the workday.

This all makes sense for those whose occupations require little physical activity, but what about those who have very physical jobs? Why are they just as susceptible to straining and having difficulty performing activities? For so many, the idea of having a physical job is considered to be the answer to keeping muscles strong and balanced. When I have treated people who have had neck or back pain or pain at an extremity, they often seemed confused when I said the cause was muscular. Many tell me, "But I do physical work all day. Doesn't this keep my muscles strong? How can I possibly be straining muscles when they are working so hard as a result of what I do all day?"

While performing physical activity every day does maintain muscles that have already been strengthened and are balanced, to live a life free of pain, *all* the muscles required must be strong and balanced. If they aren't, one or more muscles will strain and elicit pain or lead to altered positions of joint surfaces that lead to joint pain. As such, you must perform some type of isolated progressive resistance exercise that focuses on keeping all muscles strong by isolating the individual muscles to strengthen them.

Furthermore, physical jobs often put the individual in awkward positions and still require strong muscles to create force. Let's look at a mechanic who might have to bend to get under a car or twist to get to a particular part of a motor. They might have to be on one foot while reaching to create force to tighten or pull on something. While doing these actions on two feet in a stable position might be something the muscles can perform without straining, doing it in an unstable position requires energy to go to the balance-stabilizing muscles instead of toward performing the task at hand. Awkward, unstable positioning also makes the ability to use leverage to create force more difficult. This combination of factors alters the force capacity of the muscles performing the task and can lead to straining.

Let's say you need to lift an object off the floor and put it on a table. The most effective mechanism to do this would be to stand with your feet on either side of the object and to lift the object right in front of you, pushing up equally with both legs so that each leg supports 50 percent of the load to lift the object.

Now let's think about what happens in real life. The phone is ringing, you have a bunch of other things to do, you are thinking about what you have to do after work, and without paying much attention, you lift this object. But instead of evenly distributing the weight between both legs, you lift it with one side of the body. This means that one leg will have to lift 80 to 90 percent of the load while the other leg is mostly helping to maintain your balance. Without even remotely realizing it, you just strained your back or the knee or hip muscles. Pain occurs in the overstrained leg, but with your busy life, you may not realize it until the next morning when it is hard to get out of bed due to the pain. If you had conditioned all your muscles to be strong and balanced, the strength of the muscles of the legs and torso would have been able to absorb this increased force and would have prevented the strain.

Fig. 3-5a. Lifting with both legs

Fig. 3-5b. Lifting with one leg

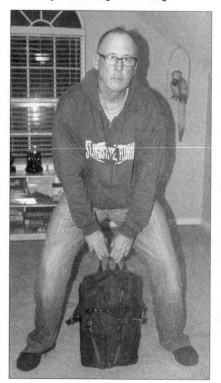
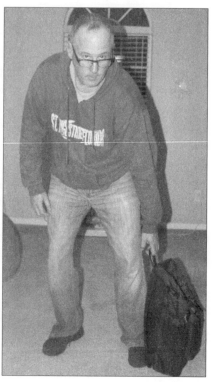

Whether or not we like it, the truth is that life moves quickly. You won't always have time to make sure you do everything mechanically correctly, and some jobs simply require dealing with awkward, strenuous forces. The only solution is to develop strong, balanced muscles to ensure that you can handle whatever life throws at you without straining weakened or inactive muscles.

CARRYING

Many people carry a bag over one shoulder or, in the case of a clutch or a briefcase, sometimes hold it in one hand. That load is being supported by only one of two sides of the body. You have two arms and two legs for a reason. They are designed to break loads up to 50 percent on one side and 50 percent on the other. Carrying shoulder-style bags on one side unwittingly creates a load that will pull you toward that side, resulting in muscles on the other side of the body being forced to contract in a way that is not efficient, and may result in pain in unlikely areas. For example, carrying your pocketbook on the left shoulder can cause you to end up with right neck or lower back pain. Backpacks or similar carrying bags are designed to distribute the weight more easily and can mitigate this sort of imbalanced straining.

The muscles of the hip and knee can also feel the effects of imbalanced strains. A heavy load being carried on the left shoulder will cause you to bend to the right side to try to offset the excess load. This means you will be putting more weight on the right leg, which will in turn make the muscles of the right hip and knee work harder than the left hip and knee. You'll end up getting pain in the right hip or knee region from strained muscles, which may again cause you some confusion. The problem here is that the cause of the pain is an alteration of forces. Since forces are invisible, it may be the primary reason that many never think them to be the cause of pain.

Now that you know why pain can develop, you can take a very simple step to prevent your neck, back, hip, and knee regions from experiencing pain without seeking unnecessary medical care. If there is one lesson you can take from me, it is that every bit of evidence proves that the cause of most pain is due to muscle strain and associated compensations. The cause in most cases is weakness or imbalance of muscle and altered forces due to the way activities are performed, which heighten the force requirements of certain muscles that are not designed to take these loads. The answer, my friends, is to simply control and prepare for the forces that are thrust upon us in our daily lives.

Beyond paying attention to how we carry what we carry, the best way to prevent strain is to strengthen all the muscles associated with carrying. Here is another place where my information may differ from the normal advice. Typically you are told to strengthen all your muscles equally, front to back, top to bottom. Before doing so, you must consider that most everything you do is performed in front of the body. This leads to natural muscle imbalances. The chest, front shoulder, and front upper arm muscles are generally stronger than the muscles between the shoulder blades, back shoulder, and back of the upper arm. This leads the shoulders to be drawn forward and the head to hang forward. Strengthening of all the muscles, including the chest and biceps, will actually sustain this imbalance, exacerbate improper posture, and lead to strain and pain at the neck and upper back.

Therefore, I highly recommend starting a strength-training program by only strengthening the muscles of the upper back, back shoulder, and back upper arm. This will achieve a healthy posture and strengthen all the muscles that are involved in supporting the arms and any objects that are held or carried. The muscles to be strengthened are the posterior deltoid, the rhomboids, the mid-traps, the lower trapezius, the rotator cuff, and the triceps. The exercises to be performed are posterior deltoids, lat pulldown with neutral bar, lower trap, external rotation, and tricep extension. Strengthening of the forearm extensors (muscles on the top of the forearm) will help to keep the forearm flexors (muscles that help to grasp and hold objects) from excessively shortening and straining leading to pain at the inner elbow or even creating carpal tunnel syndrome (the real cause).

➤ **Posterior Deltoids:** *Gorilla Arms*

See p. 191 for instructions.

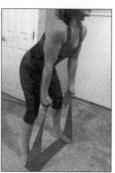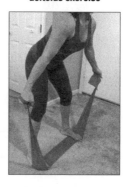

Fig. 3-6a. Beginning of posterior deltoids exercise

Fig. 3-6b. End of posterior deltoids exercise

➤ **Lat Pulldown with Neutral Bar:** *Pull Down from Shelf*

See p. 190 for instructions.

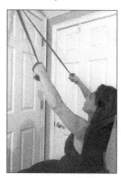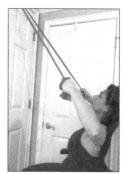

Fig. 3-7a. Beginning of lat pulldown

Fig. 3-7b. End of lat pulldown

➤ **Lower Trap:** *Paint the Wall*

See p. 190 for instructions.

**Fig. 3-8a. Beginning of
lower trap exercise**

**Fig. 3-8b. End of lower
trap exercise**

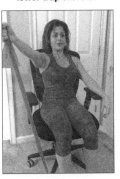 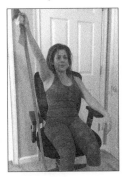

➤ **External Rotation:** *Reverse Hammering*

See p. 188 for instructions.

**Fig. 3-9a. Beginning
of external rotation**

**Fig. 3-9b. End of
external rotation**

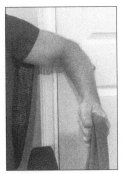 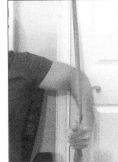

➤ **Tricep Extensions:** *Casting a Fishing Rod*

See p. 193 for instructions.

Fig. 3-10a. Beginning of tricep extensions

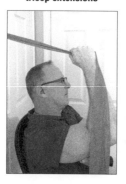

Fig. 3-10b. End of tricep extensions

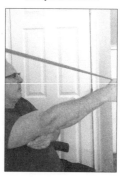

➤ **Wrist Extension:** *Raising Back of Hand*

Strengthens the forearm extensors

Means of resistance: dumbbell or resistance band

Place the forearm on the leg with the wrist hanging in front of the knee and the palm facing down. Place the opposite hand on the top of the forearm to keep it stable and prevent it from raising during the exercise. Start with the hand face down. Bend the wrist upward raising the hand as high as it can go. Then return to the start position.

Fig. 3-11a. Beginning of wrist extension

Fig. 3-11b. End of wrist extension

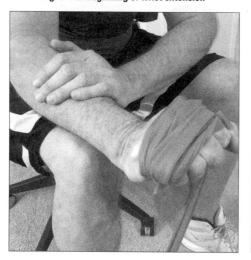

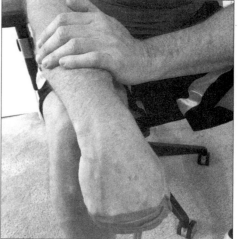

LIFTING

Most of us are familiar with the advice that you should lift with your legs. That is only half true. You do want to lift with your legs, but you should also maintain a slight arch in your lower back. Not doing so is the primary reason people get back pain when they lift objects. Many people have been told not to arch their back as a general rule, and the advice generally rings true. Having an excessive arch in the lower back is a sign that the hip flexors and front thigh muscles are too short and too strong in relationship to the opposing muscles, the gluteus maximus muscle and the hamstrings, which can lead to strain and pain. A mild arch is the norm for the lower back. However, the more substantial arch from lifting an object plays a role in the way the forces transmit through the lumbar spine.

In looking at the anatomy of the spine, there is a little protuberance on the top of the back of the vertebrae that sticks up above a little recess. When the lower back is arched, the protuberance moves into the recess and the vertebrae become locked. It is called a facet lock. This is critical for force to transmit through the spine, as now you no longer have five independent vertebrae but one continuous one. This allows force to run through the spine very effectively, protecting the structures of the spine, but, most importantly, taking so much of the load as to not force the muscles of the lower back to overwork. Lifting with a rounded back prevents the facet lock from occurring, and the spine will not take much load at all. The majority of the forces are then absorbed by the lower back muscles, which are not designed to take these loads. They were designed to simply transmit weight from the torso to the legs. This is what leads to straining of the lower back when the right technique is not used.

So now that you will arch your back when lifting objects to prevent strain and pain, let's talk about how you should use your legs. The primary way to lift an object is through the squat movement.

Fig. 3-12a. Beginning of squat

Fig. 3-12b. End of squat

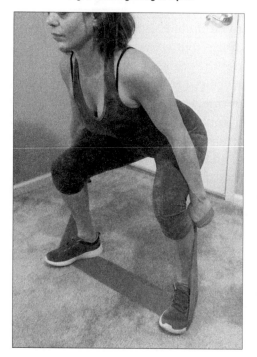
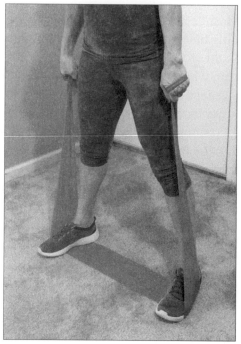

With this movement, you lift with the quads (the front thigh muscles). These are the biggest muscles of the body and are therefore best designed for lifting. But here is the next big pitfall: most people think a squat and a deep knee bend are the same thing, but they are not. A deep knee bend is when you move toward the ground with your shoulders, hips, and ankles all in alignment. A squat movement requires that the shoulders, *knees*, and ankles are in alignment.

Fig. 3-13. Deep knee bend

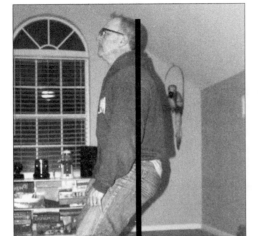

Fig. 3-14. Proper squat

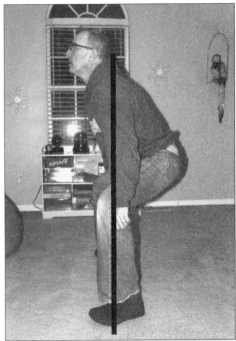

Since the knees stay over the ankles while squatting, the shin is maintained in an almost vertical position. The quad muscle is actually attached to the kneecap, which is attached to the lower leg bone by a tendon. This means that the quad creates force and lifts you by pushing off the lower leg bone. It has the best ability to create force when the lower leg bone is fully erect. Therefore, the squat is the most advantageous way to lift objects. Squat with your back slightly arched while holding the object you are lifting as close to you as possible, and you will be able to lift the heaviest object you can in the most effective manner with the least chance of strain and pain.

Here's another key point: since the quads are the primary muscle responsible for lifting in a squat movement, the natural inclination is to believe that you need to strengthen your quads. Not so fast! Remember when I mentioned that there are certain predisposed muscle imbalances? This is the biggest one in the body. Most people have much stronger quads than hamstrings. This means the quads will have a tendency to shorten. If you strengthen them in this shortened state, they will shorten further, leading to straining and eliciting pain at the back, thigh, or knee. To test if this is the case, attempt to perform a quad stretch. (See p. 208 for instructions.)

Fig. 3-15. Quad stretch

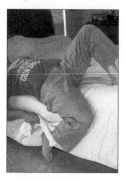

If you can bring your heel to your butt, you can strengthen your quads with knee extensions, lunges, or squats and feel confident that these exercises will help you lift objects with greater ease. (See p. 199 for instructions.)

Fig. 3-16a. Beginning of knee extension **Fig. 3-16b. End of knee extension**

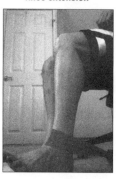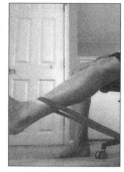

Fig. 3-13. Deep knee bend

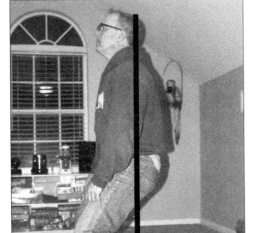

Fig. 3-14. Proper squat

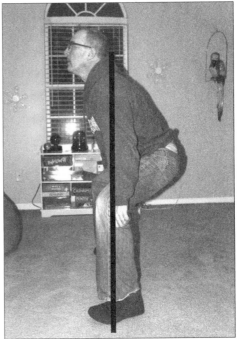

Since the knees stay over the ankles while squatting, the shin is maintained in an almost vertical position. The quad muscle is actually attached to the kneecap, which is attached to the lower leg bone by a tendon. This means that the quad creates force and lifts you by pushing off the lower leg bone. It has the best ability to create force when the lower leg bone is fully erect. Therefore, the squat is the most advantageous way to lift objects. Squat with your back slightly arched while holding the object you are lifting as close to you as possible, and you will be able to lift the heaviest object you can in the most effective manner with the least chance of strain and pain.

Here's another key point: since the quads are the primary muscle responsible for lifting in a squat movement, the natural inclination is to believe that you need to strengthen your quads. Not so fast! Remember when I mentioned that there are certain predisposed muscle imbalances? This is the biggest one in the body. Most people have much stronger quads than hamstrings. This means the quads will have a tendency to shorten. If you strengthen them in this shortened state, they will shorten further, leading to straining and eliciting pain at the back, thigh, or knee. To test if this is the case, attempt to perform a quad stretch. (See p. 208 for instructions.)

Fig. 3-15. Quad stretch

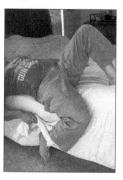

If you can bring your heel to your butt, you can strengthen your quads with knee extensions, lunges, or squats and feel confident that these exercises will help you lift objects with greater ease. (See p. 199 for instructions.)

Fig. 3-16a. Beginning of knee extension **Fig. 3-16b. End of knee extension**

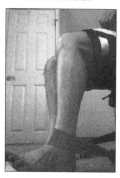 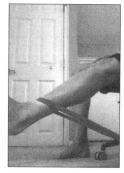

➤ **Lunges:** *Single-Leg Kneel*

Strengthens the quads

Means of resistance: dumbbells or resistance band

Lunges require a bit of balance to complete, so please don't do them if you feel unsteady in any way. You might want to perform this exercise without using extra weight (so you can grab on to something during the motion); however, using resistance in each hand will improve your balance because the weight on either side of your body will help to stabilize you. To do this exercise, spread your feet a little wider than shoulder width apart. Then place one foot in front of you and one foot behind, keeping them the same width apart. The whole foot of the front leg should be on the floor, while only the balls of the foot of the leg behind should be on the floor. Next, lower the back knee toward the floor. The front knee will bend, but make sure it does not end up in front of the front foot. Lower yourself until the front thigh is parallel to the floor. Then return to the start position. Keep the torso upright during the whole motion. The back leg should feel like it is just there for balance. The ability to lower and raise yourself should feel like it is coming from the front foot—that is, you should feel like you are pushing primarily through the heel of the front foot.

Fig. 3-17a. Beginning of single-leg kneel   **Fig. 3-17b. End of single-leg kneel**

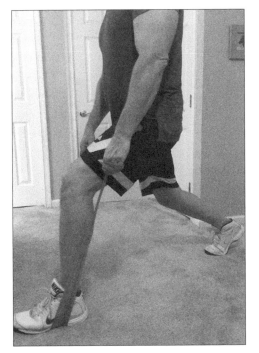
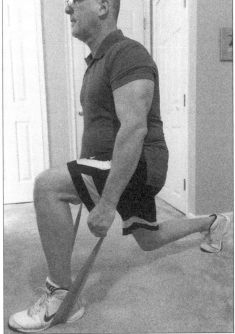

➤ Squats: *Sit Down/Stand Back Up*

Strengthens the quads primarily

Means of resistance: dumbbells or resistance band

The main muscle that performs the squat is the quads (front thigh muscle), not the hamstrings or butt muscles. To perform the squat, start with your feet a little more than shoulder width apart and your toes pointed outward. The knees should be unlocked with the butt pushed backward slightly. Hold the resistance in your hands, with your hands at the side of the body. The key to performing a squat properly is to envision that you are sitting down in a chair. The butt should move backward as the shoulders move forward. The knees should remain as close to over the ankles as possible. Remember that a deep knee bend is when you go down and the knee moves forward but the hips stay over the ankles. In a squat the knees stay over the ankles and the butt goes backward as the shoulders move forward. The goal is to sit down far enough until your thighs are parallel to the ground, and then return to the start position. For some, balance might be an issue. If so, don't go too far down. As you gain confidence and strength, you can work your way to the point where your thighs are parallel to the ground. You can also put a chair behind you. This will not only help you visualize the idea of sitting down in a chair; it will also catch you if you lose your balance.

Fig. 3-18a. Beginning of squats

Fig. 3-18b. End of squats

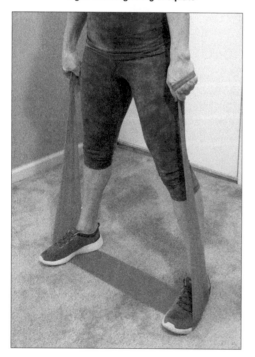

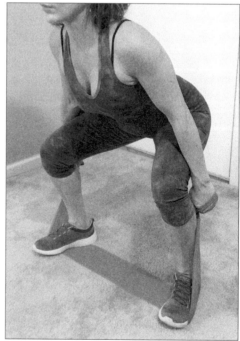

If you cannot bring your heel to your butt, your quads are too strong and you need to strengthen the hamstrings to help lengthen your quads to their optimal length. Begin with the quad stretch, hamstring curl, hip extension, and straight leg deadlifts until the heel can be brought to the butt, and then add in the quad exercises. (See pp. 208, 196, 198, and 204 for instructions.)

Fig. 3-19. Quad stretch

Fig. 3-20a. Beginning of hamstring curl

Fig. 3-20b. End of hamstring curl

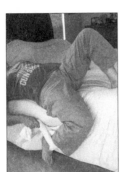
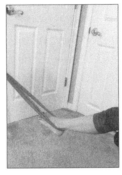
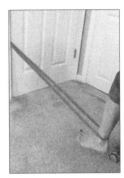

Fig. 3-21a. Beginning of straight leg deadlifts

Fig. 3-21b. End of straight leg deadlifts

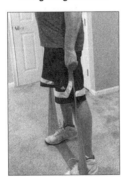
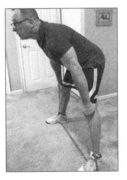

Let's briefly talk about lifting from waist height to shoulder height or above. The first bit of advice is to try to lift the object centered between your legs. This gives you the best chance to use all the muscles on both sides of the body and equally disperse the forces developed from lifting the object. Next, consider what is the best way to position your torso. If you are lifting an object that is held in front of you, the load will likely cause you to lean forward. Instead of simply allowing this force to be absorbed by muscles of the upper back and arms, try to let your spine take some of the load. Lean back slightly when standing, which is achieved by activating the hips with the gluteus maximus and hamstring muscles. By leaning back, the force is moved from in front of the hips to over the hips. This makes the load more easily supported. The only force being created is the one to lean back and that is being achieved by muscles designed to achieve this goal. If lifting over shoulder height, this leaning back posture helps to keep the load over the hips, limiting any load in front of the body that would have to be picked up by muscles not designed to take this load. If you are placing an object on a shelf at waist height or above, get as close as you absolutely can to the shelf. Any distance between you and the shelf increases the distance away from your legs, and thus increases the amount the load will have to be supported as it is placed on the shelf. It is not simply the weight of the object that determines the forces that are created and need to be supported—it is also the distance away from the body that the object must be supported.

In terms of lifting objects from waist height to shoulder height and above, the muscles that create hip extension or leaning back (the hamstrings and gluteus maximus) are key. These can be strengthened by performing hamstring curls, hip extensions, and straight leg deadlifts. (See pp. 196, 198, and 204 for instructions.)

**Fig. 3-22a. Beginning
of hamstring curl**

**Fig. 3-22b. End
of hamstring curl**

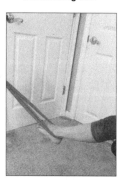
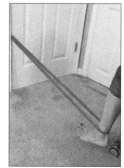

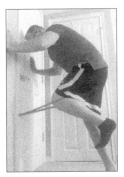

Fig. 3-23a. Beginning of hip extension

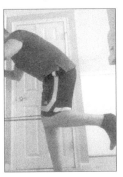

Fig. 3-23b. End of hip extension

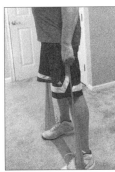

Fig. 3-24a. Beginning of straight leg deadlifts

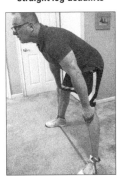

Fig. 3-24b. End of straight leg deadlifts

For the upper body, strengthening of the muscles of the upper back, posterior shoulder, and triceps is key. To do so, try the lat pulldown with neutral bar, lower trap, posterior delt, external rotation, and tricep extension. (See pp. 190, 191, 188, and 193 for instructions.)

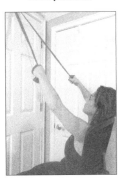

Fig. 3-25a. Beginning of lat pulldown

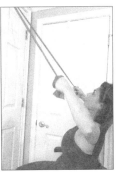

Fig. 3-25b. End of lat pulldown

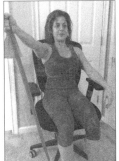

Fig. 3-26a. Beginning of lower trap exercise

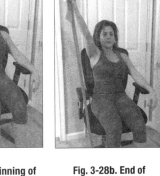

Fig. 3-26b. End of lower trap exercise

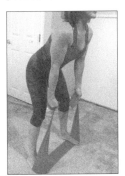

Fig. 3-27a. Beginning of posterior deltoids exercise

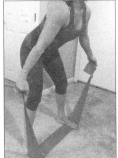

Fig. 3-27b. End of posterior deltoids exercise

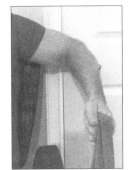

Fig. 3-28a. Beginning of external rotation

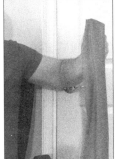

Fig. 3-28b. End of external rotation

Fig. 3-29a. Beginning of tricep extensions

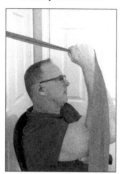

Fig. 3-29b. End of tricep extensions

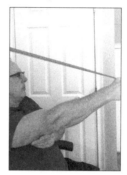

ON THE PHONE

In terms of spending lengthy periods of time on the phone, technology has certainly helped decrease the need for what was often a recipe for neck pain and headaches. People had the tendency to hold the handset of the phone against their ear by lodging it on their shoulder. This would lead to the muscles of the upper back and neck working excessively hard to support the handset, which would lead to strain and pain. Now there are headsets that hook into the telephone system or computer for hands-free use. If you have moved to this type of system, that's great. If not, I would highly recommend getting one of these devices. If a cell phone is used at work, Bluetooth-connected headsets can also prevent the need to hold the phone up to the ear with your hand, where the weight of the arm has to be supported for an extensive period of time, in turn leading to strain and pain. The first line of defense in being able to work with maximum productivity with the least chance of straining and eliciting pain is the strengthening and balancing of your muscular system. Beyond this, mechanical changes that can alter the forces that might be required to be absorbed by muscles should be an important part of your strategy to get the most out of your body while at work.

ON THE COMPUTER

Despite what we typically think of as strenuous jobs, such as those that pertain to heavy loads or awkward positions, other types of seemingly subdued jobs should also be considered strenuous. Occupations such as secretaries, paralegals, computer programmers, or any other job that requires large amounts of computer use and typing should be considered strenuous activities. It may not necessarily be for the whole body, but certainly is the case for the upper body since you are supporting your arms for eight to ten hours a day in order to type. Your arms possess a good deal of weight running from the shoulder and shoulder blade complex to your rib cage and your primary skeleton. The average person that performs these types of jobs ends up leaning forward with their head bent forward and down, causing strained neck and upper back muscles, as well as migraine headaches.

I try to encourage people who perform what seems like simple activities that span several hours a day to think of themselves as athletes. Everybody accepts the idea that athletes need to train and condition themselves for the sport they are going to play. You too must condition yourself for the activity you are going to perform. If typing is a major required portion of your job, strengthen every part of the upper back muscles and muscles that support the shoulder blade against the rib cage. Strengthening the posterior shoulder muscles, the rotator cuff, and the muscles between the shoulder blades and the back of the arm will support the arms and create a better posture, allowing you to hold your head upright over your shoulders. The exercises for these muscles include posterior deltoids, lat pulldown with neutral bar (rhomboids/mid-traps), lower trap (lower trapezius), external rotation (rotator cuff), and tricep extension (triceps). (See pp. 191, 190, 188, and 193 for instructions.)

Fig. 3-30a. Beginning of posterior deltoids exercise

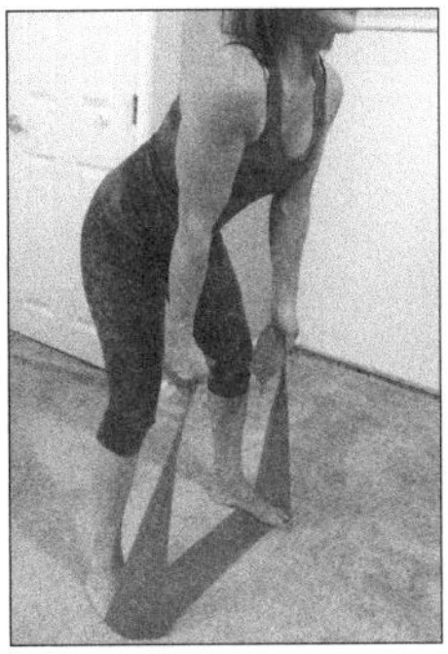

Fig. 3-30b. End of posterior deltoids exercise

Fig. 3-31a. Beginning of lat pulldown

Fig. 3-31b. End of lat pulldown

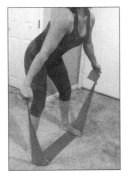
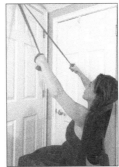
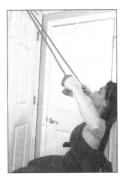

Fig. 3-32a. Beginning of lower trap exercise

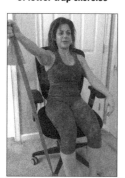

Fig. 3-32b. End of lower trap exercise

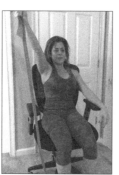

Fig. 3-33a. Beginning of external rotation

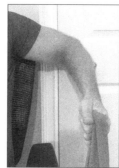

Fig. 3-33b. End of lower external rotation

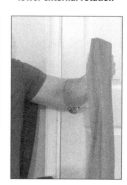

Fig. 3-34a. Beginning of tricep extentions

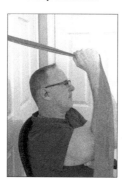

Fig. 3-34b. End of tricep extentions

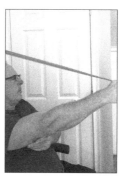

One tip beyond muscle strengthening is to get forearm supports for your desk or to set the keyboard and mouse such that your arms are supported on the desk. Set the height of the monitor to allow you to look straight ahead, and set your chair so that your back is supported. If you were to look at your profile posture, your shoulders should be just behind your hips.

Fig. 3-36a. Shoulders just behind hips

Fig. 3-36b. Shoulders in front of hips

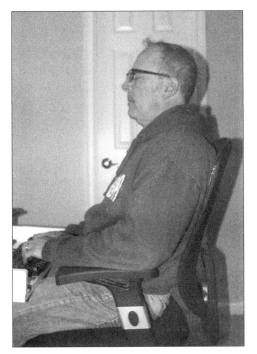 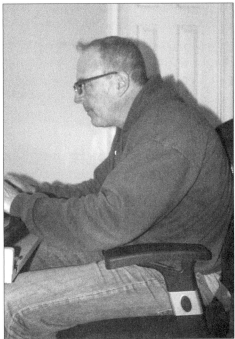

This will help to stop the natural progression toward developing forward shoulder posture and stop the need to support the head by the muscles of the upper back. Working on a computer does not have to lead to neck pain, upper back pain, or headaches. Take the right steps and do the right exercises to allow yourself to be optimally productive with the least chance of injury.

YOUR COMMUTE TO WORK

Driving is the way that many people travel to work. The commute can be a time where business is integrated into the ride, or perhaps it is a time to eat or call a loved one. Stress associated with the coming day's trials and tribulations might have you amped up a bit, which can lead to your muscles contracting and possibly straining at a time when you wouldn't expect strain to occur.

One way to minimize physical strain during the commute is to set your seat to maximize support and limit overuse of your muscles. Putting the back of the seat to directly upright may instinctively seem like the most efficient position, but this is actually not true. Since your body has some girth, having the seat straight upright will cause your body to slightly lean forward. This means the muscles of the lower back will have to work to support the torso and prevent it from leaning forward. Your hip flexors are actually shortened in this position, especially when the angle between the torso and the leg is less than 90 degrees. A fully upright position also makes your hip flexors more susceptible to straining and spasming. The strained hip flexors can create centralized lower back pain.

The best and most efficient position for the seat back is about 10 degrees behind straight upright. This causes the upper body to lean backward very slightly, allowing the force of the torso to move backward against the seat back so the seat back will support the torso without making any demands on the muscles. With regard to the legs, keep the seat far enough from the pedals to prevent the knee from being at a 90-degree bend or fully straightened. Either position can lead to muscles being too shortened or lengthened for a sustained time, which can lead to straining. Most people think that straining can only come from a muscle overworking, but severely shortening or stretching a muscle for a sustained period of time can also be a cause of strain. Muscles like the hamstrings and the ITB band are highly susceptible to straining from overstretching or lengthening caused by the position of the knee when driving for sustained periods of time. If you have a long commute, stopping intermittently and getting out and stretching can also help to prevent your muscles from stressing in the long-sitting time frame.

Fig. 3-37. Optimal position for driving

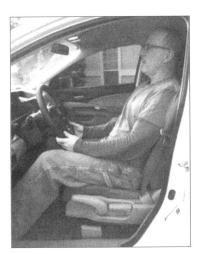

WORKING AT HOME

Working at home can lead to the problems related to inactivity because the person doesn't have to leave home to get to their workplace. Walking or stair climbing might not be necessary when working at home, and chances are high that sitting takes up a large portion of the day. As in the previous cases of sedentary work, when an activity of some force requirement is needed, muscles that have weakened and diminished in force output will become susceptible to straining and eliciting pain.

My recommendation for people who work from home is to incorporate breaks in the day where both isolated strength training can be performed as well as other types of physical activity, such as walking or climbing stairs. Since the person is at home, even activities like gardening or other household projects would fit the bill for sustaining strength and balance of muscle, accompanied by, of course, a targeted isolated strength-training program.

CHAPTER FOUR

At Play and Physical Fitness

WARMING UP

Most people, I believe, have the sense that jumping into a basketball game or starting a match of tennis doesn't make sense without warming up first. However, I'm not sure if people think about why and how warming up limits the chances of injury and developing pain. When you are lying down or sitting, the body is not working too hard. Muscles are not being used a lot. As a result, there is a low degree of lactic acid being developed. As you now know, lactic acid develops as a by-product of muscle contraction and has the capacity to cause the pH of the blood to become too acidic. This is bad for the body. So the body has a desire to bring the lactic acid to the liver for processing and removal. This is what causes increased blood flow to go to where muscles are being used. The blood is warm, so it has a tendency to cause muscles to become more lengthened and stretched out, which will help prevent straining of excessively shortened muscles.

Now let's say you have to travel by car to where you are going to play your game or participate in a fitness activity. You sit before you begin. This means that there is a strong likelihood that your muscles are not at their optimal length and thus are more susceptible to straining. It also means that they will have greater difficulty in creating the force required to perform the activity.

If the right thing to do before beginning a sport or fitness activity is to warm up, then what do you need to do exactly? Most people feel that stretching is the key. I rather take the opinion that anything that can help warm up the muscles is a good start. So a bit of a walk or a light jog would fit the bill here. Get the muscles working a little bit and lactic acid will begin to develop, leading to increased circulation to the muscles, which will warm them up. Truthfully, it doesn't take much. A couple of minutes of minimal to moderate movement should be all it takes to have those muscles ready to go. Just remember that fitness and sports activities are ballistic in nature, meaning that there is a lot of stop and go associated with the activity. The force creation of the muscles involved is much greater than just moving joints through a range of motion, so you will need to make sure your muscles are warm and ready to produce this type of force and motion.

STRETCHING—IS IT ALWAYS NECESSARY?

There has been a longstanding battle about when stretching should be performed—before performing an activity, after, or both? Let's first talk about the value of stretching, which should help answer this question. There is a sense that when a muscle is shortened, stretching is the key to lengthening the muscle. However, frequently a muscle is shortened because its opposing muscle is not as strong. As a result, the tone of the affected muscle is greater than the opposing muscle.

While stretching helps to lengthen muscles in the short term, how does it change the force equation between the two muscles? For example, your quads, or front thigh muscles, are stronger than your hamstrings, or posterior thigh muscles. Say your quads are always shortened and tight. You can try to stretch them, which in the short term will help to give them more length, but because of the imbalance of strength between the quads and hamstrings, the force output of the quads will always be greater than the force output of the hamstrings. To resolve the shortening of the quads for good, you need to strengthen the hamstrings, which can be accomplished by performing hamstring curls or straight leg deadlifts.

The false view that stretching lengthens muscles always worries me since it is only a very short-term mechanism. Let's say you've stretched your quads and are going to play a game or sporting event. Once you begin, the quads' increased force output will still overcome the hamstrings' weaker output, making the quads susceptible to straining despite the warm-up stretching. Thus, for the purpose of warming up, I always recommend moving enough to get lactic acid developing and blood flowing into muscles.

Now what about stretching after the activity? *This* is when I would recommend it. Regardless of the activity performed, the mere use of muscle is going to cause it to shorten, even with balanced muscles. Lengthening them out at the end of an activity brings them back to their optimal length and allows them to sustain that length once the activity has ended. Stretching and warming up need to be seen as distinct practices with separate purposes and benefits.

DOING TOO MUCH OR TOO LITTLE

When engaging in a sport or fitness activity, the goal is to have fun and enjoy yourself. It is a chance to break away from the daily grind that we all find ourselves caught up in. From a physical perspective, it is a chance to activate your muscles. As previously stated, moving and performing activity by itself does not achieve strength and balance. It does, however, sustain strength and therefore limits the potential for atrophy, strain, and painful symptoms. To know if you are working your muscles enough to sustain their strength, it is advisable to use an exertion scale, which can help determine if you are getting enough out of the activity. Think of a scale from 0 to 10. Zero feels like you are doing nothing, and 10 feels like you are going to tear a muscle. Try to participate at an exertion level around 7 or 8. This means you are using 70 to 80 percent of your maximum effort. This is a good level to ensure that you're getting value from performing the activity without worrying about straining and injuring yourself.

When it comes to strength training, I am always astounded when I see people at the gym talking to their neighbor, reading an article, or watching television while supposedly engaging in strength training, particularly when they later go on to express surprise or dismay about not getting any value from the exercise. An old rule holds true: you get out of something what you put into it. If you are strength training and you can focus on something other than the strength training, then you are certainly not exerting the appropriate level of energy to maximally benefit from your efforts.

Fitness activities are your chance to make sure you are keeping your muscles strong enough to perform the tasks of daily living like walking, negotiating stairs, bending, kneeling, reaching, or lifting. However, when we undertake these activities, we are more likely to be doing too much than too little. We all watch our favorite players perform at the highest level, and we wish to perform with similar levels of talent and capacity. What you never see is the countless hours they put into conditioning their bodies so that when they perform with such high levels of exertion, their bodies are ready. Their muscular strength and balance allow them to create optimal force and perform at their greatest function.

Don't push yourself beyond your body's capacity to perform. Be in tune with your body. If you begin to experience pain when performing a fitness or sports activity, stop and analyze the situation. Pain is a sign that a tissue is in distress and should not be ignored. Being in the heat of the moment with your adrenaline pumping tends to make you feel like you can do a lot more than what your body can really achieve. Try not to overdo it, as you will have to pay for it later.

TAKING A BREAK

Part of listening to your body involves knowing when it is time to take a break. When adrenaline is flowing, it is harder to hear the messages being sent from the body. Carbohydrates typically fuel the performance of sport or fitness activities. These types of activities are considered anaerobic, which means that not enough oxygen is being taken in while performing them. As a result, fat cannot be used as the fuel source. Carbohydrates create half the energy that fat can when broken down (four calories per gram of carbohydrates versus nine calories per gram of fat). Because there is a tendency to burn through these calories at a fairly swift pace, an intermittent break while performing sports is a good idea. You can regain some energy by eating fruit or an energy bar that can be readily digested. Drinking water and replacing electrolytes is also important. Blood is 90 percent water, so if you are performing a fitness activity or participating in a sport and sweating a lot, it is important to replace the fluid that is lost. When you sweat, you also lose electrolytes that are key for muscle contraction, including from the heart. One point of note is that during breaks, try not to completely cool down. You want to maintain blood flow into the muscles to keep them warm and at their optimal length.

Breaks should be built into the regimen of the game or sport. Intermittent breaks are key to sustaining maximal performance and preventing against injury. Don't wait until you get dizzy or feel lightheaded. Don't wait until it feels difficult to bear weight. You can see this in just about any sport played professionally, and you should be no different. Just think about the fact that if injury occurs while playing a sport or participating in a fitness activity, it will affect all aspects of your life.

THE MYTH OF GIVING UP WHAT YOU LOVE

As I have mentioned earlier, one of the worst adages of the medical establishment is *if it hurts, don't do it*. I have met way too many people who were told that they need to give up golf or tennis because it led to shoulder, back, knee, hip, or ankle pain. As far as I am concerned, the professional is acknowledging that they don't know what is causing the pain being experienced, so their only option is to tell their patients not to do the thing causing the pain. This is a very sad precedent, not to mention an entirely unnecessary one. Pain is an indication of a tissue in distress. The goal of medical professionals should be to identify the tissue and find a way to resolve distress, which will eventually stop the tissue from needing to create the pain signal. Pain does not exist on its own. Fix the tissue, and end the need for the pain signal.

For example, if tennis causes shoulder pain, it is because it is an activity in which the tissue being affected and creating the pain signal is muscle. You need to figure out which muscles are straining. Strengthen or balance the responsible muscles, and you will have pain-free tennis. If you have back pain or knee pain from playing golf, the same principles apply. Figure out which muscles are not working properly, achieve balance and strength of the pertinent muscles, and you can play as much golf as you would like.

Because muscular causes of pain, such as strains or imbalances, cannot be identified by MRI diagnostic tests and there is no medical specialty educated or designed to identify them, you are basically held prisoner to the existing system. Which is to say that you are always being told the cause of the pain is a structural variation that can only be resolved through surgery. You are then left with the choice to risk surgery with the evidence pointing to it failing in most cases or to simply stop doing what you love.

But you don't have only two choices. You have a third. Use the Yass Method to identify whether the tissue eliciting your pain is muscle, and if so, establish what needs to be strengthened or balanced to get yourself back to doing what you love. Not being able to do what you love should not be a consequence of an inept system.

The lower back plays an integral role in most activities, particularly recreational ones. When lower back pain arises, the natural tendency is to assume it is from the spine. If you seek medical attention, a diagnostic test might find a structural abnormality and there you have it: the decision to quit the sport or get surgery.

The first thing you must know is that the spine is not as fragile as the medical establishment would have you believe. It is not easily injured with the awkward movement or increased force required by sports or fitness activities. The lower back is supported by the lower back muscles, called the quadratus lumborum.

Fig. 4-1. Quadratus lumborum

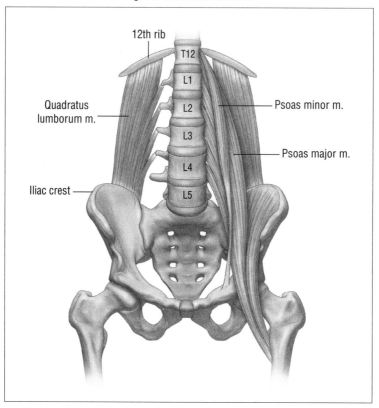

These muscles run from the underside of the rib cage to the top of the pelvis. The length of the muscles determines how much force they can create and how well they can perform their functional responsibility of supporting the torso. The relationship between the quads and hamstrings determines what the length of the lower back muscles will be. Since the quads attach to the front of the pelvis and the hamstrings attach to the back of the pelvis, the lengths will determine how close or far away the pelvis will be from the bottom of the rib cage. If, as in most cases, the quads are stronger than the hamstrings, the quads will shorten and pull the front of the pelvis down, causing the back of the pelvis to rise and move closer to the bottom of the rib cage. The lower back muscles may then shorten, strain, and emit pain. From a functional standpoint, this also prevents both side-bending and the rotation of the torso from being performed at their optimal range. Resolution of this issue can be achieved by stretching the quads and strengthening the hamstrings and gluteus maximus. The exercises to be performed are the quad stretch, hamstring curl, and hip extension. (See pp. 208, 196, and 198 for instructions.)

Fig. 4-2. Quad stretch

Fig. 4-3a. Beginning of hamstring curl

Fig. 4-3b. End of hamstring curl

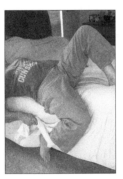
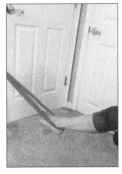
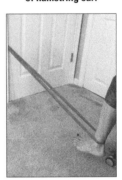

Fig. 4-4a. Beginning of hip extension

Fig. 4-4b. End of hip extension

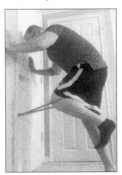
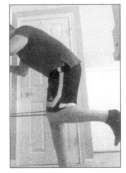

On the other hand, if hamstrings are stronger and shorter, then the back of the pelvis will be pulled down and the lower back muscles will be lengthened. This condition would reveal itself as a flattened lower back, causing the lower back muscles to overstretch and strain. Here you would want to stretch the hamstrings and strengthen the quads. The exercises to be performed are hamstring stretch, knee extension, and squats. (See pp. 206, 199, and 202 for instructions.)

Fig. 4-5. Hamstring stretch   **Fig. 4-6a. Beginning of knee extension**   **Fig. 4-6b. End of knee extension**

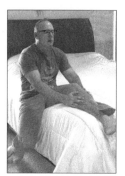
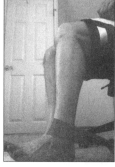
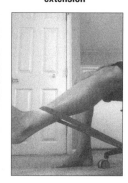

Fig. 4-7a. Beginning of squats   **Fig. 4-7b. End of squats**

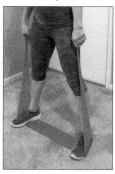
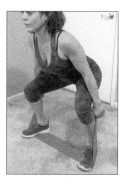

If you want your lower back muscles to perform optimally and you want to maximize your lower back flexibility, the key is to achieve balance of the quads and hamstrings. Forget the concept of the "core." There is no basis for the idea that the abdominal muscles assist with back stability. Strengthening the lower back muscles will reinforce a natural imbalance between the lower back muscles and abdominal muscles, causing you to arch your lower back excessively, which will lead to back pain and the loss of flexibility.

The other imbalance that needs to be addressed at the lower back is between the hip flexors and gluteus maximus. The psoas portion of the hip flexors actually attach to all five lumbar spine vertebrae. When shortened, your back can feel like it is being pulled into your stomach. If lower abdominal pain is felt at the same time as lower back pain, it is actually a reinforcing symptom, indicating that the cause is shortened and strained hip flexors. Pain from this type of issue would be experienced close to the lumbar spine rather than the lower back. Difficulty standing upright is another indicator of this imbalance. The functional deficit is the same as shortened lower back muscles: a severe loss of lower back flexibility. Stretching of the hip flexors and strengthening of the gluteus maximus and hamstrings will resolve this deficit and maximize the functional capacity of the lower back. The exercises to be performed are the hip flexor stretch, hamstring curl, and hip extension. (See pp. 206, 196, and 198 for instructions.)

Fig. 4-8. Hip flexor stretch

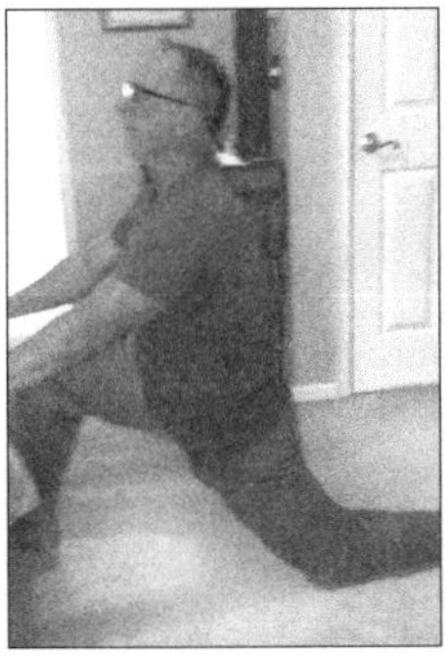

Fig. 4-9a. Beginning of hamstring curl

Fig. 4-9b. End of hamstring curl

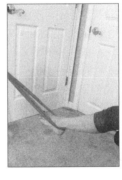
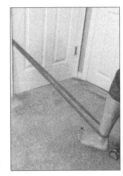

Fig. 4-10a. Beginning of hip extension

Fig. 4-10b. End of hip extension

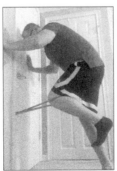
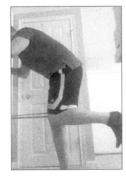

Your lower back is key to performing fitness or sports activities without injury. Maintaining balanced muscles will keep the lower back at its most optimal posture, allowing you to perform at your highest level.

ARE YOU A WEEKEND WARRIOR?

How many people sit at a desk all day during the week and then decide they are an NFL quarterback, an NBA basketball player, or a world champion tennis player on the weekend? Sports are plastered on the television screen—it's natural to dream of emulating your favorite sports stars. The sad reality, however, is that you are simply not them. High-level athletes put as much effort and time into physically training as they do mastering their sport. They have trainers and coaches making sure they get the best nutrients to maximize their performance. If you have a job where you sit most of the day and have trouble getting your three square meals in, your body will not be able to meet your brain's expectations of what you can do.

This is not to say that you should give up playing your favorite sport on the weekend. It is simply to say that you should take a lesson from the very players you look up to. If you want to perform strenuous activities on the weekend, then you are going to have to condition yourself during the week. What most people do not understand is that many of the aspects of weekday activities are the very causes of injury and pain on the weekend. The number one culprit for the source of strain is the natural imbalance that occurs from sitting long stretches of time. As a general rule, most people have a muscle imbalance between the quads and hip flexors versus the gluteus maximus and the hamstrings because we usually move forward to perform activities. Sitting and standing, walking, negotiating stairs, and kneeling all occur in front of us, making high demands from the hip flexors and quads. Because of this imbalance, the hip flexors and quads will have a tendency to shorten. For some, this shortening can become extensive.

When it's time to get up for lunch or to go home, you may have a massive amount of pain at the lower back, the knees, or both. You can't stand upright because of the back pain and you can't straighten your knees out. This indicates that something is wrong with how your muscles are functioning. Yet when the weekend comes, do you then decide it is okay to go full throttle and perform sporting activities with severe forces and aggressive movements, and expect nothing to happen? Not so fast, my friend.

A simple thing to do to help condition yourself is to work to maintain balance between the hip flexors and quads versus the gluteus maximus and hamstrings. It is your best chance of minimizing back and knee pain. To achieve this goal, perform hip flexor and quad stretches, as well as hamstring curls, hip extensions, and straight leg deadlifts. (See pp. 206, 208, 196, 198, and 204 for instructions.)

Fig. 4-11. Quad stretch **Fig. 4-12. Hip flexor stretch** **Fig. 4-13a. Beginning of hamstring curl** **Fig. 4-13b. End of hamstring curl**

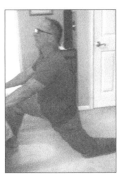 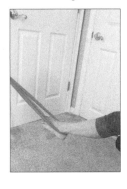 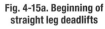 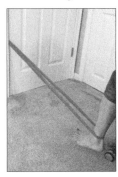

Fig. 4-14a. Beginning of hip extension **Fig. 4-14b. End of hip extension** **Fig. 4-15a. Beginning of straight leg deadlifts** **Fig. 4-15b. End of straight leg deadlifts**

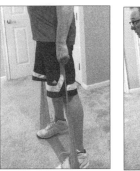 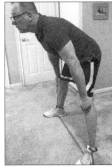

The next thing you can do to maximize your weekend sport fest without ending up calling in sick on Monday is to strengthen the gluteus medius muscles. These are the muscles that sit just above the hip joint. They are responsible for creating balance and stability during single-leg standing. They are designed to stabilize the pelvis so muscles attached to the pelvis like the quads and hamstrings can pull off to create maximal force and allow quick movements. The gluteus medius are the muscles that create movement in the legs. If they are weak, you will be more unstable and the muscles that move you will have a more difficult time creating their force, which in turn will make it harder to perform vigorous activities. To achieve optimal strength of the gluteus medius muscles, perform hip abductions. (See p. 196 for instructions.)

Fig. 4-16a. Beginning of hip abduction exercise

Fig. 4-16b. End of hip abduction exercise

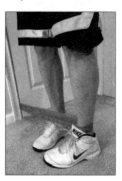
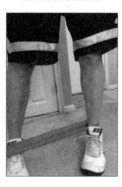

Fig. 4-16c. Beginning of hip abduction exercise

Fig. 4-16d. End of hip abduction exercise

Fig. 4-16e. Side view of hip abduction exercise

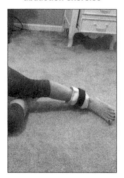
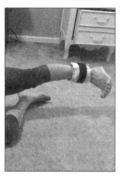
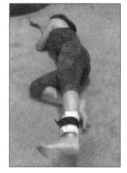

With regard to the upper body, to prevent against shoulder injuries, mid-back or neck pain, or even headaches, you will need to address the typical imbalance that exists between the pecs, the front shoulder, and bicep muscles, versus the muscles between the shoulder blades, the back shoulder, and triceps. This imbalance has a tendency to cause the shoulders and head to be drawn forward. The muscles that support the shoulder, shoulder blade, and the head will then become overstretched and susceptible to straining. This area of muscles also includes the rotator cuff, which is a critical muscle for any type of shoulder function. The number of muscles involved in the use of the arm is much greater than the leg because of the complexity of how the shoulder and shoulder blade function. The muscles that should be strengthened to maximize balance and function of the upper body are the posterior deltoids, rhomboids/mid-traps, lower trap, rotator cuff, and triceps. The exercises to be performed are the posterior deltoids, lat pull-down with neutral bar, lower trap, external rotation, and tricep extension. (See pp. 191, 190, 190, 188, and 193 for instructions.)

Fig. 4-17a. Beginning of posterior deltoids exercise

Fig. 4-17b. End of posterior deltoids exercise

Fig. 4-18a. Beginning of lat pulldown

Fig. 4-18b. End of lat pulldown

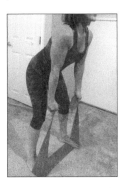
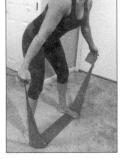
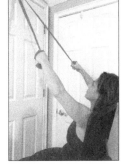
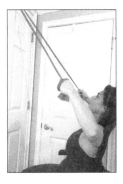

Fig. 4-19a. Beginning of lower trap exercise

Fig. 4-19b. End of lower trap exercise

Fig. 4-20a. Beginning of external rotation

Fig. 4-20b. End of external rotation

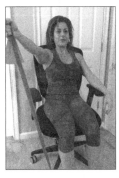
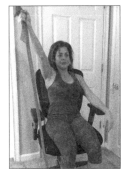
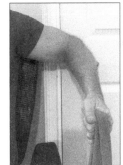
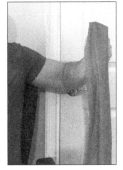

Fig. 4-21a. Beginning of tricep extensions

Fig. 4-21b. End of tricep extensions

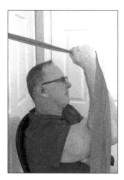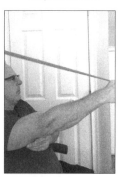

You have to be realistic about playing sports on the weekend when you spend most of your weekdays sitting at work. Just as you must recognize this fact, I must recognize that you only have so much time during the week to give to strength training. That is why I have designed a minimalist method to get the most out of your effort. I suggest strengthening only the muscles that are most apt to lead to injury and lack of maximal performance. These muscles just need to be strengthened three times a week. The key is to optimize your resistance in order to perform the exercises and develop enough strength to have a great time on the weekend, as well as hopefully minimizing your chances of being carted off the field on a stretcher.

TAKING UP A NEW SPORT

The idea of taking up a new sport is a fabulous and exciting venture. It stimulates both the mind and the body. A new sport requires new movement patterns to be developed. Coordination and balance, as well as athleticism, will be challenged in new ways. This, in turn, helps new nerve pathways develop in the brain, which is great for brain health. Force requirements may be different from anything attempted before. All of these are reasons to take it slow when starting a new sport. I would recommend learning the basic elements of the sport first and practicing these before getting into a full-blown game.

If you are taking on tennis, for instance, go to a park and start out by hitting a ball against a wall. If basketball is your choice, practice dribbling and shooting before entering a game. For golf, go to a range and practice swinging with different clubs before heading out on the course. All of these activities have a component of momentum built into them, meaning that speed will be involved. Muscles must be trained to handle this type of load. Strength training should be performed at a controlled and uniform speed to allow the muscles to adapt to the resistance and ultimately get stronger. On the other hand, with sports, quick movements and development of speed are key to increasing the movement of a racket or a club. Therefore, muscles will be lengthened or shortened much faster, making them much more susceptible to straining and creating pain. So general strength training should be performed in a slow and controlled manner to allow muscles to adapt and get stronger, while sports-specific training should employ ballistic types of movement to condition the stronger muscles to be able to react more quickly.

A combination of strength training during the week to prepare your muscles and practicing the individual elements of the sport to allow the muscles to adapt to the new speed requirements will perfectly prepare you for picking up a new sport and having the most fun on the weekend, which we all deserve after a long, grinding week.

UNDERSTANDING YOUR LIMITS

Just because you see somebody perform something at a high level does not mean you can (or should) do it too. Innate talent plays a key role in performing well, and this might be something you simply don't have. However, let me be clear that I am vehemently against the idea that age plays a critical role in the ability to participate in sports. The biggest determinant is a person's physical condition. The question is whether you have prepared yourself to participate in a sport so that you can perform at *your own* best level while limiting your chance of injury. Remember that you must train and condition yourself during the week if you plan on participating in sports on the weekend. You also have to be realistic about what you can and can't do in terms of your talent capacity. Play at a level where you feel challenged, but not at a level where injury is more prevalent or frustration will develop because you are in over your head.

I am a huge fan of challenging myself, but there is no question that satisfaction comes from winning as well. These two aspects of playing sports should be considered when deciding to what extent you plan to challenge yourself and at what level of competition you choose to participate. If you are just starting a sport, give yourself some time to learn what has to be done at the beginner level and give yourself the leeway to get good there before entering competition. Try to have fun, challenge yourself, and be safe all at the same time.

CHAPTER FIVE

Sleeping and Relaxation

WHY PAIN OCCURS AT NIGHT

One of the biggest issues that confuses people about their pain is why it is worst during the night or when they wake up. This actually indicates that a muscle is responsible for the pain. To understand why, we need to revisit how lactic acid build-up affects the lengh of muscle. When muscles are being used during the course of the day, lactic acid develops. Lactic acid is a by-product of muscular contraction. Lactic acid being acidic can alter the pH of the blood. This can be dangerous for the body, so the lactic acid must be drained from the muscles and brought to the liver to be broken down. This means that an increase in blood is flowing to your muscles when you are active. The good thing about this occurrence is that blood is warm. With the excess warm blood flowing to your muscles, they have a tendency to remain lengthened. Since pain receptors run through the connective tissue of muscle fibers, the lengthened muscle means that pain receptors are maintained at a longer distance apart. This reduced concentration of pain receptors results in less pain experienced.

At night, however, when you are recumbent, there is little movement, which means that limited amounts of lactic acid develop. If no excess blood is sent to the muscles, the muscles will be maintained at a cooler temperature. If the muscles have strained or if there is an imbalance, they may tend to remain shortened. This means that a much higher concentration of pain receptors can develop, making pain more likely to be experienced.

Many people have their worst shoulder pain at night. They might describe pain near the shoulder or even an altered sensation running down the arm or the hand going numb when they lie or sleep on their side. This is not confusing or surprising when you understand how the rotator cuff works and why this position can stress this muscle group. The rotator cuff attaches from the shoulder blade and surrounds the head of the upper arm bone as it sits in the shoulder joint.

Fig. 5-1. Roator cuff

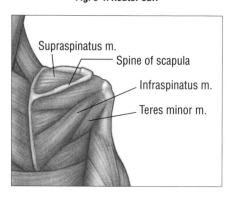

When strong and fully functional, the rotator cuff keeps the head of the upper arm bone centered in the shoulder joint. If strained and weakened, it finds this difficult to achieve. When you lie on your shoulder while sleeping on your side, all the pressure of your body can fall on the shoulder. The arm bone will have a tendency to slide forward if it is not maintained in the center of the shoulder joint. This movement will move the arm bone farther away from the shoulder blade, creating stress and pain on the rotator cuff because it becomes overstretched. Muscles and nerves have a capacity to create and transfer symptoms such that the strained rotator cuff might refer altered sensation down the arm and cause the hand to feel numb. This might be enough to wake you up. Usually if you turn over or shake the arm, the symptoms quickly resolve, but your sleep will have been affected. The key to preventing this from happening is to keep the rotator cuff and surrounding shoulder and shoulder blade muscles strong and balanced.

Another common way to irritate the rotator cuff into straining and either eliciting pain at the shoulder or referring symptoms down the arm is sleeping with your arm pointing up with your head lying against the arm. Sometimes people find it more comfortable to lay their head on their arm when sleeping rather than against a pillow. This is another position where the rotator cuff can become overstretched and strained.

Fig. 5-2. Person sleeping with head on arm

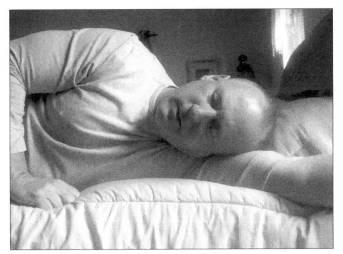

An important point to make is that not only are muscles prone to strain when supporting a load greater than the force output of the muscle, but they can also strain if overstretched or shortened, as they often are while we sleep.

A common fear when waking up at night from having altered sensation or numbness at the hand is the assumption that some neurological distress may be at fault. As a general rule, it is more likely to be muscular in nature, which is why shaking or moving the limb with the symptoms will often quickly resolve it.

Those who experience knee pain at night most often have a muscle imbalance between the front thigh muscles and the back thigh muscles. The front thigh muscles, the quads, have a tendency to become stronger than the back thigh muscles, the hamstrings. This causes the quads to shorten. Remember that at night, with no activity being performed, muscles will obtain their shortest lengths. If you sleep on your side in a fetal position, your knees will be bent to somewhere around 90 degrees, causing the quads to be shortened substantially. Since the quads attach to the kneecap by a tendon, the shortened length of the quads will have a tendency to pull the kneecap into the knee joint with much greater force, causing it to be compressed in the joint.

Fig. 5-3. Quads attaching to kneecap

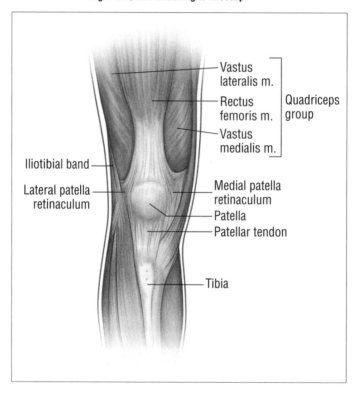

When you suddenly decide to move or get up from the bed, the movement of the joint or the weight bearing on the joint can create severe pain. You can prevent this situation by keeping the quads lengthened and balanced to their opposing muscles, the hamstrings. To achieve this goal, perform the quad stretch and hamstring curl. (See pp. 208 and 196 for instructions.)

Another reason for knee pain at night is a shortened and strained ITB band, the connective tissue band that runs from the pelvis down the side of the thigh to the knee.

Fig. 5-4. ITB

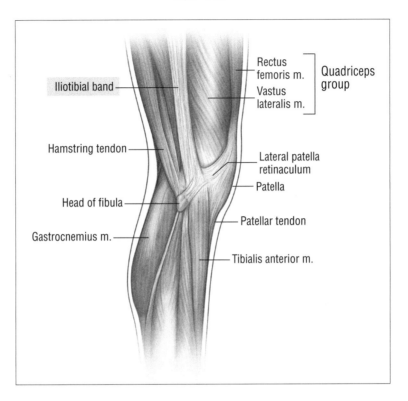

If strained and irritated, it will pull the kneecap laterally, causing the kneecap to impact the lateral border of the knee joint. In a fetal position or position where the knee is bent for a sustained period of time, the ITB will have a tendency to shorten. When you suddenly try to straighten your knee, as when you stand up from the bed, massive compressive forces between the kneecap and the lateral border of the knee joint can cause a good deal of pain. Even if you have your knee bent for a period of time and are simply trying to adjust your position in bed, straightening your knee can cause pain at the knee joint. The ITB and the muscle that is attached to it at the top, called the tensor fascia lata, can become irritated and strained if the muscle that sits just above the hip joint, the gluteus medius, strains first. This muscle provides balance and stability when single-leg standing. Keeping the gluteus medius muscle strong—along with other muscles, such as the gluteus maximus and hamstrings that work in conjunction with it—will prevent it from straining and leading to the ITB straining and shortening. To achieve this goal, perform the ITB stretch, hip abduction, knee extension, and hip extension. (See pp. 207, 196, 199, and 198 for instructions.)

Neck pain while sleeping or at night may occur on just one side of the neck or across both sides. If it is only on one side, you most likely have a problem with the muscles that perform shoulder function. This might seem at odds with logic, since the pain appears to be at the neck region, but the neck and the shoulder are connected. The levator scapulae, a muscle that runs from the upper cervical spine to the shoulder blade, also runs through the area called the upper trap region.

Fig. 5-5. Levator scapulae

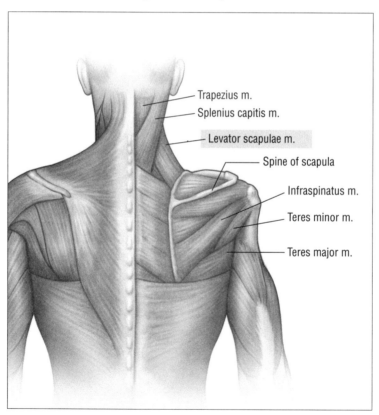

Right now when you feel neck pain, you probably press on the cervical part of the neck and run your hand along the upper trap region to the shoulder. This is where this muscle exists.

The Latin name of the muscle means to "elevate the shoulder blade," and the function of this muscle is to raise the shoulder blade but to also stabilize the shoulder blade against the rib cage. Muscles attach from the arm bone to the shoulder blade, which facilitates movement in the shoulder. The shoulder blade must be held against the rib cage for this to work properly. The levator scapulae is also responsible for this function, so if any of the other muscles connected to this function strain and weaken, it can cause the levator scapulae to overwork and strain as well.

At night, the muscle will have a tendency to shorten. If the head is not maintained in its proper alignment while being held straight up, which is almost impossible to do at night when you are sleeping, the muscle can become either excessively stretched or shortened. This will lead to pain at the upper trap region into the neck. If the muscle strains enough, it might go into spasm, where you will feel like you can't move your neck at all. The way to prevent this issue is to make sure that all the muscles involved in shoulder function are kept strong and balanced. This includes the rhomboids and mid-traps, posterior deltoids, rotator cuff, lower trapezius, and triceps. The exercises to strengthen these muscles include the lat pulldown with neutral bar, posterior deltoids, external rotation, lower trap, and tricep extension. (See pp. 190, 191, 188, and 193 for instructions.)

If the pain is across both sides of the neck, you probably have a muscle imbalance between the pecs (chest muscles), front shoulder, and bicep (front upper arm) muscles versus the muscles between the shoulder blades, posterior shoulder, and triceps (back upper arm). This imbalance is a natural occurrence resulting from the fact that we perform all tasks in front of us. This means with everything lifted, held, or manipulated in front of us, the chest, anterior deltoid, and biceps are used much more than the muscles between the shoulder blades, posterior deltoids, and triceps. When this imbalance increases, the shoulders will move forward and the shoulder blades move farther away from the spine. Any muscle that attaches from the spine to the shoulder blade can become overstretched. The levator scapulae muscle attaches from the upper cervical spine to the upper inner corner of the shoulder blade, meaning that the muscle will be overstretched in this altered posture. When the muscle becomes overstretched, it loses its ability to perform one of its functional tasks, which is to support the head. It will have a tendency to shorten when strained. So at night, when it is not used, it is going to be given its chance to shorten excessively. Even if you keep your head perfectly upright and not bent to one side or the other, the excessive pull of the strained levator scapulae will still elicit pain at both sides of the neck.

The issue here, believe it or not, is typically how many pillows are in use. The problem isn't whether the head is bent sideways, but how much space exists between the chest and the chin. Either too much forward bending of the head or too much extending of the head backward can cause the levator scapulae to elicit pain at the neck region. To prevent this from occurring at night, maintain balance between the chest, front shoulder, and biceps versus the muscles between the shoulder blades, posterior deltoids, and triceps. Strengthening of the muscles of the upper back and back of the upper arm will prevent the muscles, including the pecs, from shortening and creating the altered posture of forward shoulder.

Certainly one of the bigger symptoms people feel at night is sciatica. This is when you have pain or an altered sensation from the gluteal region down the leg past the knee, most often to the foot. This can be a debilitating pain and has the tendency to wake you or keep you from sleeping. The most important thing to understand about sciatica is that it is not coming from the lumbar spine. In fact, it has nothing to do with the spine at all.

Fig. 5-6. Sciatic nerve with nerve roots

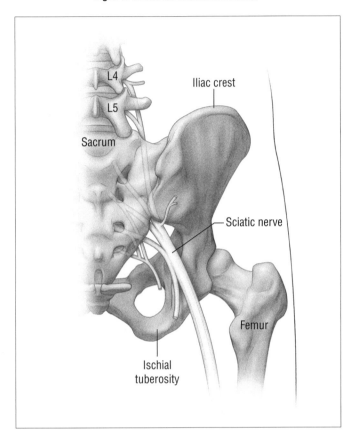

Sciatica is a hip dysfunction issue, meaning that it relates to the hip, not the back. The straining of a muscle called the gluteus medius that sits just above the hip joint on the side of the pelvis is at fault. This muscle is responsible for supporting you and giving you stability, especially with single-leg standing. When this muscle strains, the muscle that sits adjacent to it in the gluteal region, called the piriformis muscle, will try to help and compensate. Once this muscle strains, it can thicken and impinge on the sciatic nerve as it passes through the gluteal region next to and, in some cases, through the piriformis muscle.

Fig. 5-7. Piriformis muscle and sciatic nerve

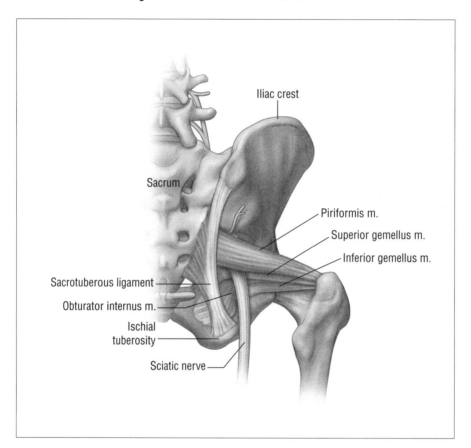

The big news here is that you have a muscular cause creating a neurological symptom. Simple ways to diminish the symptom include icing your gluteal region. Using ice for 10 minutes every hour will cause the nerve impulse to stop setting off. Stretching your piriformis is another way to take pressure off the nerve from the strained and tight muscle. The key is to strengthen the gluteus medius muscle and other muscles that work in conjunction with it to keep it from straining and to prevent the piriformis from having to try to compensate, which also leads it to straining and thickening. The muscles that need to be strengthened are the gluteus medius, quads, gluteus maximus, and anterior tibialis. Once the symptoms are concentrated in the gluteal region rather than farther down the leg, switch to just strengthening the gluteus medius, gluteus maximus, and hamstrings. The exercises include hip abduction, knee extension, hip extension, and dorsiflexion and then switching to hip abduction, hamstring curl, hip extension, and straight leg deadlifts. (See pp. 196, 199, 198, and 195, and then 196, 198, and 204 for instructions.)

Spoiler alert: the "clam shell" exercise is worthless and accomplishes nothing. Only strengthening of the appropriate muscles by performing the proper exercise with proper form and using progressive resistance will ever be able to resolve these symptoms and causes.

For those just having pain in the gluteal region at night, cause is the same as sciatica but just to a lesser degree. Most likely, the gluteus medius strained and the piriformis tried to compensate but strained as well. The piriformis strain is less significant, so it is not impinging on the sciatic nerve. Therefore, the resolution is to simply strengthen the gluteus medius, gluteus maximus, and hamstrings by performing hip abduction, hamstring curl, hip extension, and straight leg dead-lifts. (See pp. 196, 198, and 204 for instructions.)

Pain at the groin is another common complaint, and it can also coincide with pain at the hip joint region or pelvic region. The natural inclination to believe that this pain is associated with the hip joint and osteoarthritis is unfounded.

By now we know that muscles have a tendency to want to shorten when not being used, so let's see which muscles are involved in this situation. The primary muscle that can strain and elicit pain in the groin region is the sartorius muscle. It is a muscle that runs from the pelvis along the inner thigh to the inner knee. It tends to strain when the muscle that sits just above the hip joint and provides support and stability, the gluteus medius, strains first. The gluteus medius straining will create a tendency for the sartorius to shorten. At night when less blood is flowing into the muscle, it will try to shorten excessively. This is a very long muscle, so it can shorten substantially. It can cause pain in the groin region and even down the inner knee. Having this pain and pain when lying on your side at the hip region and outer pelvis are strong signs that the gluteus medius has strained. To prevent this problem from occurring, strengthen the gluteus medius, quads, and gluteus maximus and lengthen the sartorius muscle. The exercises to be performed are the hip abduction, knee extension, hip extension, and sartorius exercise.

Some people will develop severe pain at the underside of the foot near the heel at night, and the first step down on the floor in the morning can send shock waves through their body. This is a surprising phenomenon, as it comes so unexpectedly. But the reality is that there is a problem that is lurking, waiting to present itself with horrible pain. The plantar fascia is a thick connective tissue band that runs from the balls of the feet to the heel. It helps to support the arch, along with certain other muscles, and allows the foot to support the weight of the body when it is stood upon. When the muscles that help to support the arch strain, more force is created on the plantar fascia and this can irritate it. When you're inactive at night with excess blood circulating throughout the body, the plantar fascia can shorten. Since it is made of connective tissue, there are a lot of pain receptors in the tissue. When the tissue is shortened, the concentration of pain receptors increases, and when force is applied, the pain receptors ignite. The key to preventing pain from developing at the underside of the foot and heel at night is to maintain strength of the muscles responsible for helping to support the foot and arch. Keeping the gluteus medius and anterior and posterior tibialis muscles strong will stop the plantar fascia from shortening and eliciting pain with the very first step out of bed. The exercises to be performed are hip abduction, dorsiflexion, and inversion. (See pp. 196, 195, and 199 for instructions.)

A less common but possibly scarier phenomenon is being awoken with difficulty breathing and tightness and/or pain under the arms. I have treated people who experienced this and who assumed they were having a heart attack. They went to the hospital, and when everything checked out fine, they were told they were having an anxiety attack. This was confusing, as these people were not anxious types. Upon evaluation, I was able to determine that they had strained their serratus anterior muscle. This is a muscle that attaches to the underside of the shoulder blade on one side and attaches to eight ribs on the other side, and it is susceptible to the same potential for straining when shortened. This muscle may shorten to the point where it impedes the rib cage's ability to expand and contract, which is required for normal breathing. Thus, the person will find it difficult to breathe normally. Lying down also removes gravity's ability to assist the diaphragm in taking a breath. As a result, the person will wake up with difficulty breathing. This sensation, combined with pain under the arm from the muscle straining, will convince the person they are having a heart attack. To prevent this from occurring, strengthen the muscles of the upper back, including the muscles between the shoulder blades, the rotator cuff, posterior deltoids, lower trapezius, and triceps. The exercises to be performed are the lat pulldown with neutral bar, external rotation, posterior delt exercise, lower trap exercise, and tricep extension. (See pp. 190, 188, 191, 190, and 193 for instructions.)

WHY SLEEP MATTERS TO YOUR MUSCLES

Let's face it, life can be a grind. You have a lot to do in just one day. The focus of life is on completing tasks and activities, not on how you accomplish them. That is why your muscles need to perform optimally so you must keep them strong, balanced, and properly nourished. This is where sleep plays a pivotal role.

When you sleep, you allow your muscles to rest—although muscles don't ever really completely relax. Muscles are always contracting slightly in something called resting tone, which occurs even while we're asleep. While muscles contract, in addition to lactic acid, they develop waste products called metabolites. These are noxious and can hurt the performance of muscles. While we sleep, blood has a chance to run through the muscle and help wash away the metabolites, improving function and performance.

Over the course of the day, you may overwork your muscles, causing the body to pump excessive amounts of fluid into the muscle to help heal it and resulting in an inflammatory response. This is when a muscle typically feels very sore. Giving the muscle a chance to shut down at night when you sleep while the inflammatory response is in progress helps to speed up the healing of the muscle.

All cells of the body require oxygen and glucose to exist and live. Sleep provides the chance for the body to provide these nutrients to the muscles unimpeded. This can be said for all tissues of the body. The brain needs time to rest and refuel. Getting good quality sleep helps to keep the mind sharp and acute. The connection between brain function and performance is also well documented. If your mind is not at optimal performance, the ability of complex movement patterns necessary for normal daily activity might be slower and less accurate. The lack of brain control over your muscles can actually lead to overuse of muscles, putting them in danger of being strained. So getting a good night's sleep doesn't just affect the health of the muscles themselves, but also affects the health of your brain, which controls how your muscles will be used.

There are four general pillars of fitness that I try to live by to maximize my performance:

1. Exercise

2. Nutrition

3. Sleep

4. Stress reduction

All of these play a role in how efficient we will be in performing our tasks and activities. Any lack in one of these areas can lead to poor performance or injury. Most people who know me know about my obsession with strength training. But even I will admit that these four pillars are equally important to each other in achieving optimal health and optimal performance.

WHAT CAN YOU DO ABOUT IT?

Everybody is searching for the answer to relieving the pain that disrupts sleep at night. Companies sell mattresses and beds that run in the tens of thousands of dollars. There are the pillow salesmen. And there are the nutrition junkies selling natural supplements. You can certainly get lost in the barrage of products being sold.

I am constantly asked about these products and my answer is always the same: How do these products change the circumstances that are leading to pain at night or lack of sleep? In most cases, the pain is stemming from a muscle weakness or imbalance allowing a muscle to shorten excessively, causing a concentration of pain receptors to develop and emit pain. For most of the commercial products, like special pillows, there is no guarantee you will even use them as intended because you may keep your pillow between your legs or under your knees, or continuously adjust the pillow's position under your head throughout the night. The expensive beds and mattresses seem like quite a dramatic gamble, and if they don't work, you may absorb a potentially multithousand-dollar loss.

My recommendation is to focus on the cause of this nighttime dilemma, namely muscle weakness or imbalance. As mentioned earlier, in addition to resolving the muscle weakness or imbalance creating this circumstance, the next best thing you can do is to artificially bring heat to the distressed muscles. There are many manufacturers of adhesive patches that contain camphor or menthol. These types of materials create targeted heat and cause increased blood flow, which helps to warm up the muscles and keep them stretched out. You can take a hot shower before bed, but obviously there is a point at which you will begin to cool down without the heat continually being applied. You will likely find heating pads to be more effective.

One other suggestion is to try stretching before going to sleep. Stretching is a way to lengthen the muscle in a short-term manner. The only way to resolve shortening in the long term is to resolve muscle imbalances. But if you are mainly interested in short-term relief at night, stretching should be performed lightly before bed. Hold each stretch for 20 seconds, two times. These stretches should not be too intense—you should feel like if you were asked to hold it for minutes, you could. The best combination is to apply heat to your muscles first and then try a stretching regimen. To reiterate, this is just a short-term method for reducing or relieving nighttime pain while you work on strengthening muscle weakness or imbalance to resolve the pain in the long term.

BEING PROACTIVE WITH PAIN

An important lesson to take away from this book is that the pain you are experiencing at night is 100 percent the result of what you are doing during the course of your day. Overworking your muscles or being sedentary and then having to perform active tasks like walking or climbing stairs can stress muscles to the point where they strain. If you are living a fast and furious life, you probably won't let pain slow you down too much as you race through the day. But at night, you will pay the price for this type of lifestyle. You must realize that the time to address the pain you are experiencing at night is not at night, but during the day. You must recognize that the pain is the result of weakness or imbalance and the force requirements of your activities being greater than the force output of your muscles. It's not necessary to spend hours in a gym every day. Remember, the Yass Method is designed to get the most out of your time and effort. It simply calls for strengthening two to three times a week, usually taking only 45 minutes to an hour to complete.

Beyond resolving your muscular deficits, taking steps to use your muscles when you are sedentary or being careful not to strain them when using them excessively are key to preventing nighttime pain. The ways in which you support the loads you have to carry, wear supportive footwear, and adjust your seat back so the seat supports you can all play roles in how your muscles are used and how efficient you can be in your daily life.

WHEN MEDICINE MATTERS

I am certainly not a sadist, and I don't think it is right to tell somebody not to use medication ever. The idea should be to use it in the least amount and as infrequently as possible. It is important to understand that the pain being experienced is part of the distress system of the body indicating that a tissue is in distress. Medications can be used as a way of masking the symptoms. For example, sleep might be obtained with the help of medicine, but you still need to identify the tissue in distress eliciting the pain when you're trying to fall asleep so that you can resolve the issue in a long-term manner.

One type of drug that should only be used as a last resort is opioids, as they are extremely addictive and dangerous. Many people are given anti-inflammatories under the supposition that their pain is being caused by inflammation, even though the cause is more often muscular. The reason these types of drugs work is because they have a sedative effect on the brain.

Muscle relaxants are another form of medication used to address muscle pain. Relaxants can often cause fatigue, which can be positive at night, but they can also make you much less productive during the day.

I am a big fan of using natural remedies to address symptoms. So if pain is severe, try using ice on it for 10 minutes every hour. Ice is an anesthetic, meaning it blocks the transmission of pain. Heat is also great for soreness and some forms of muscle pain because it leads to vasodilation, which is an increased blood flow to the area, causing muscles to be stretched out and dispersing pain receptors that run along the muscle fibers.

If medication is something you feel you need to take, I won't try to convince you otherwise. But keep in mind that medication never addresses the actual cause of the pain being experienced—it merely offers temporary relief from the symptoms. I am a cause-and-effect guy. I will always promote that you need to address and resolve a cause to end symptoms that you experience in effect. Keep your focus on this, and your need for medication will be short-term rather than indefinite.

IS YOUR BODY TOO TIRED?

Having the ability to fall asleep on the floor, a couch, or wherever you happen to plop yourself down is a sign of being exhausted and of having an overworked body and brain. With a balanced physical and mental state, falling asleep should take 15 to 20 minutes. If you find yourself falling asleep instantly, whether you are sitting or lying down, you are probably overdoing it during the day.

The average person requires eight hours of sleep. If you are getting a full night's sleep and are still tired in the morning, it is a sign you are overdoing it. Take the time to examine *how* you are performing activities during the day. Are you not getting enough nutrition? Are you too stressed from an event in your life? Are you working way too many hours? All of these are stressors on the body. The body is amazing in its ability to be resilient, but it can only go so far before it breaks down. It is always best to try to find the stressors and resolve them before the breakdown occurs.

EXERCISES USED IN THIS CHAPTER

Fig. 5-8. Quad stretch **Fig. 5-9a. Beginning of hamstring curl** **Fig. 5-9b. End of hamstring curl** **Fig. 5-10. ITB stretch**

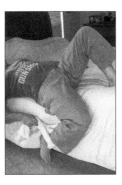 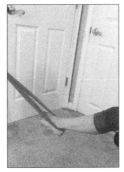 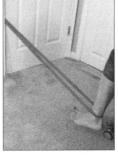 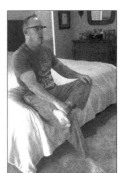

Fig. 5-11a. Beginning of hip abduction exercise **Fig. 5-11b. End of hip abduction exercise**

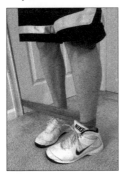 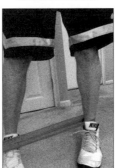

Fig. 5-11c. Beginning of hip abduction exercise

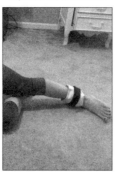

Fig. 5-11d. End of hip abduction exercise

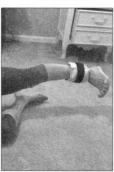

Fig. 5-11e. Side view of hip abduction exercise

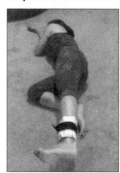

Fig. 5-12a. Beginning of knee extension

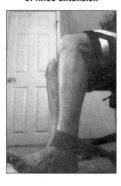

Fig. 5-12b. End of knee extension

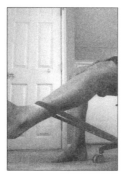

Fig. 5-13a. Beginning of hip extension

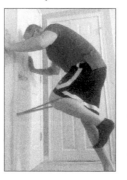

Fig. 5-13b. End of hip extension

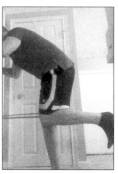

Fig. 5-14a. Beginning of lat pulldown

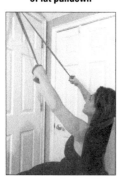

Fig. 5-14b. End of lat pulldown

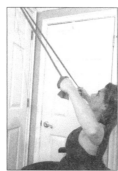

Fig. 5-15a. Beginning of posterior deltoids exercise

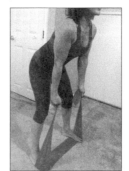

Fig. 5-15b. End of posterior deltoids exercise

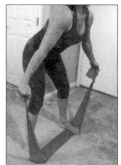

Fig. 5-16a. Beginning of external rotation

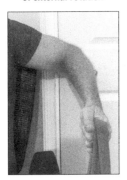

Fig. 5-16b. End of external rotation

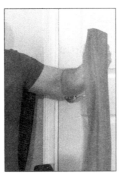

Fig. 5-17a. Beginning of lower trap exercise

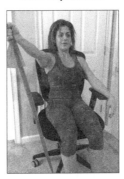

Fig. 5-17b. End of lower trap exercise

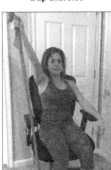

Fig. 5-18a. Beginning of tricep extensions

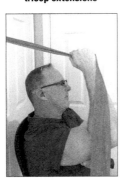

Fig. 5-18b. End of tricep extensions

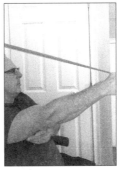

➤ Dorsiflexion: *Reverse Gas Pedal*

Strengthens the anterior tibialis

Means of resistance: machine or resistance band

With the leg supported on a surface and the ankle and foot hanging off, attach the resistance so that it is supported in the mid-foot region at the instep. Then attach the resistance between the door and frame near the bottom. You should be seated on a chair and your lower leg supported on another chair or ottoman. The key is that the foot is positioned above the height of the attachment of the band into the door to allow it to remain on the instep throughout the exercise. Start with the ankle angled about 30 degrees forward; then pull the ankle toward the face, about 10 degrees beyond perpendicular. Then return to the start position.

Fig. 5-19a. Beginning of dorsiflexion

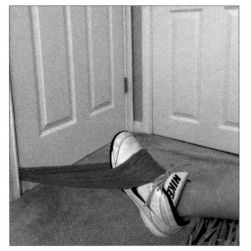

Fig. 5-19b. End of dorsiflexion

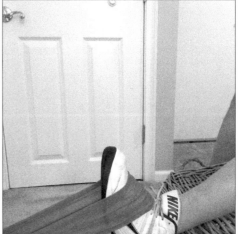

Fig. 5-16a. Beginning of external rotation

Fig. 5-16b. End of external rotation

Fig. 5-17a. Beginning of lower trap exercise

Fig. 5-17b. End of lower trap exercise

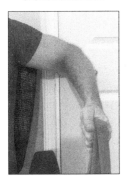

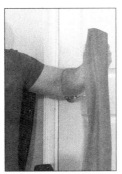

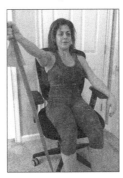

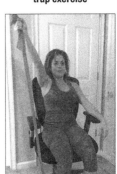

Fig. 5-18a. Beginning of tricep extensions

Fig. 5-18b. End of tricep extensions

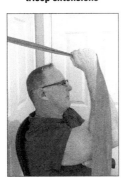

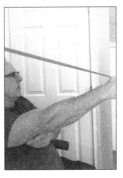

➤ **Dorsiflexion:** *Reverse Gas Pedal*

Strengthens the anterior tibialis

Means of resistance: machine or resistance band

With the leg supported on a surface and the ankle and foot hanging off, attach the resistance so that it is supported in the mid-foot region at the instep. Then attach the resistance between the door and frame near the bottom. You should be seated on a chair and your lower leg supported on another chair or ottoman. The key is that the foot is positioned above the height of the attachment of the band into the door to allow it to remain on the instep throughout the exercise. Start with the ankle angled about 30 degrees forward; then pull the ankle toward the face, about 10 degrees beyond perpendicular. Then return to the start position.

Fig. 5-19a. Beginning of dorsiflexion

Fig. 5-19b. End of dorsiflexion

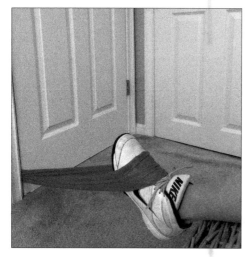
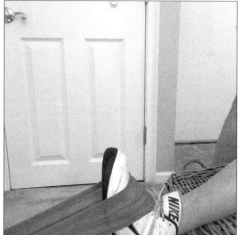

➤ **Straight Leg Deadlifts:** *Run the Hands down the Thighs*

Strengthens the gluteus maximus and hamstrings

Means of resistance: dumbbells or resistance band

Start with your feet a little more than shoulder width apart and your toes pointing slightly out. You should be standing straight with your knees unlocked and your butt pushed back slightly. Hold the resistance in front of your thighs. Bend from the hips, keeping your back straight while looking out in front of you, and begin to lower the resistance down your legs. Make sure your knees don't bend and the motion is coming from your hips. As you move down, you should feel your weight shift to your heels. When you begin to feel tightness at the back of your thighs, slowly straighten back up to the start position. There is no specific point to reach down on the leg. Reach down until you feel tightness at the back of your thighs. Make sure your back remains straight, not rounded. If it's rounded, you can strain your back and you will also go down farther than you could with a straight back. As you go down, you will feel your weight shift back onto your heels. Make sure that the resistance is held tight to your thighs throughout the whole exercise.

Fig. 5-20a. Start of straight leg deadlifts

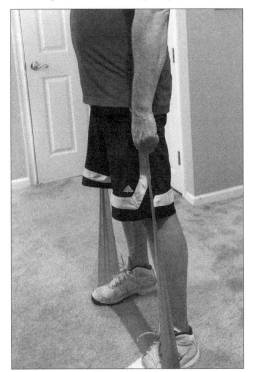

Fig. 5-20b. End of straight leg deadlifts

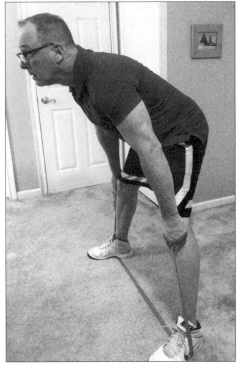

➤ **Sartorius:** *Step One Foot behind the Other*

Lengthens the sartorius muscle

Means of resistance: cable machine or resistance band

Make sure you are holding on to a sturdy object while performing this exercise to help you with your balance. In a standing position, place the resistance around the back of the ankle of the leg to be strengthened. Start with the toes of the leg that is working pointing in slightly. Then place the foot of the exercising leg behind the foot of the leg you are standing on. Once the foot of the exercising leg is placed down on the floor behind the other leg, return it to the start position. Make sure the resistance is appropriate so you can get your exercising foot behind the foot that you are standing on. You want to use a resistance that helps lengthen the sartorius, but because there is a balance element to this exercise, caution should be used in determining the right resistance. Try to keep the knee of the exercising leg straight while the knee of the leg being stood on should be unlocked. Try not to rotate the pelvis as you are performing the exercise. Both the shoulders and pelvis should be facing forward during the whole exercise.

Fig. 5-21a. Beginning of sartorius

Fig. 5-21b. End of sartorius

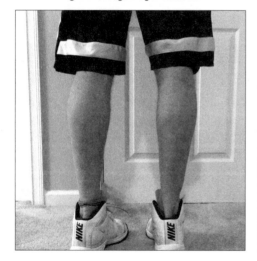
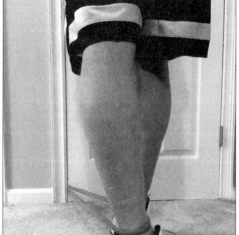

➤ **Inversion:** *Turn Foot In*

Strengthens the posterior tibialis

Means of resistance: cable machine or resistance band

Sitting in a chair, have the resistance coming from your side of the leg to be exercised (if using a resistance band/tube, place the resistance between the door and frame near the floor). Place the resistance around the instep of the foot. The heel should be on the floor with the rest of the foot above the floor. Start with the toes outside the heel and slowly pull the toes in until they are on the inside of the heel. The foot will turn upward slightly as the foot is moved inward. Then return to the start position. Place your hand on the side of the knee of the working leg and make sure it does not move. You do not want any movement or rotation of the working leg. The only motion that should be occurring is at the ankle.

Fig. 5-22a. Beginning of inversion

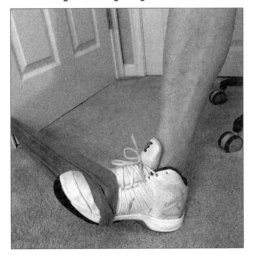

Fig. 5-22b. End of inversion

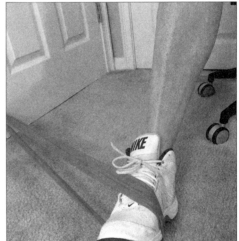

CHAPTER SIX

On the Go–from Travel to Constant Motion

SHOES, STILETTOS, SNEAKERS, AND A LEG UP ON PAIN!

How many women have been told never to wear high heels because they are bad for you? I am here to provide you with a new message. Wear your high heels as much as you want. Embrace your love of style, and feel free to express your inner beauty. That said, there are a couple of caveats, as there usually are. Wearing high heels changes the surface area that supports your body weight, increasing the forces required to keep you upright. Let's say you get to the beach and want to take a walk. If you try to walk on the sand with a flat shoe, you will have no problem traversing the ground. Now let's say you try the same thing but with a stiletto heel. What will happen? You will no longer be able to continue walking because your heel will keep digging into the sand, preventing you from moving forward.

So what changed? It wasn't the force of gravity or your own body weight, both of which remained the same. What changed was the amount of surface area supporting your body weight. In the case of the flat shoe, the weight was diffused over enough surface area that the sand was able to support you and you could therefore glide across the sand without any difficulty. In the case of the stiletto heels, your body weight was no longer being supported over the entire surface area of the foot, but only on the point of the heel. This dramatically decreased the area supporting your weight.

What if the surface were not sand, but solid? A sidewalk, for instance. The concentration of the force through the stiletto isn't picked up by the surface that you are walking on, but is moved upward to the muscles that support you. This means that your muscles are going to have to work much harder. Wearing high heels creates two kinds of increased force: side to side and front to back.

The side-to-side issue has to do with the gluteus medius muscles, which must be trained to address the increased load or force requirement of wearing high heels. These are the muscles that sit just above the hip joint on the side of the pelvis. The exercise to strengthen the gluteus medius is hip abduction. (See p. 196 for instructions.)

The key here is not to simply do the exercise, but to progress the amount of resistance used in the exercise so the muscles can get stronger. Once strong enough to take the load of being balanced on a small surface area, you are eliminating the chance for this muscle to strain and elicit pain or cause other muscles to strain by overcompensating for the gluteus medius muscle.

Now let's look at the front-to-back issue of wearing high heels. In high heels your heels are positioned much higher than the balls of your feet, which pushes your center of mass forward. You are, in a sense, forcing yourself to push your body weight onto the balls of your feet. If I were to suddenly freeze you in this position, you would clearly fall forward. This implies that an excess forward load has been created and must be absorbed by muscles in the back of the body. It could be your lower back muscles, hamstrings, or calves. You might find that you get back pain when you wear high heels, tightening at the back of the thighs, or even cramping at the calves. Sometimes these symptoms occur at night well after the day is done, where you can't immediately determine a cause for the symptoms, which may cause some confusion or anxiety.

The great news is that there is always a solution when symptoms are caused by altered forces. Train yourself to create an opposing force to the one pushing you forward in high heels. If you strengthen the gluteus maximus muscle (buttock) and hamstrings (posterior thigh), you will create a more functional hip extension. Hip extension can be visualized by thinking about the relationship between the torso and the thigh, where you extend your hip when the back of the torso is moving closer to the back of the thigh. Because the torso moves forward if you're wearing high heels, the angle between the back and the back of the thigh will increase, creating the load that may strain muscles in the back or back of the legs.

Strengthening the gluteus maximus and hamstrings will allow you to pull your torso toward the back of the thighs, helping you remain upright and diminishing strain. The exercises that need to be performed are hamstring curl, hip extension, and straight leg deadlifts. (See pp. 196, 198, and 204 for instructions.)

Again, the key is not to simply do the exercises but to continually increase the resistance being used to allow the muscles to get stronger and support you, eliminating any excess load.

There you have it! A foolproof plan to allow you to wear high heels to your heart's desire. When you are just starting this process, I would recommend taking some precautions while you build up your strength. When you are traveling, try to wear a more comfortable, flatter shoe. If you are concerned about painful symptoms that occur at night from wearing high heels, try to stretch before sleeping and use some method of heating the distressed muscles to keep them warm at night.

Beyond high heels, my general rule for footwear is that as long as the shoe is generally supportive, style should be left up to the individual. I do, however, wish there was a sensible shoe enforcement officer to tell people who live in flip-flops that this is a horrible practice and must be ended. These types of shoes are much less supportive, meaning that they are not improving your base of support when you perform weight-bearing activities. It could be said that these types of shoes actually decrease your base of support just because of how unstable they are.

However, if you do choose to wear flip-flops, it must be understood that the increased forces developed from the level of instability have to be picked up somewhere, and that somewhere is your muscles. All the muscles that support the ankle and certainly that poor gluteus medius muscle will be challenged. Strengthening these muscles will help to take the load of wearing unstable shoes and allow you to wear them for longer periods of time without jeopardizing your muscles and hurting yourself. The ankle muscles to be strengthened are the anterior and posterior tibialis muscles, along with the gluteus medius muscle. The exercises to be performed are dorsiflexion, inversion, and hip abduction. (See pp. 195, 199, and 196 for instructions.)

Just remember, for every choice you make when it comes to the shoes you wear, increased forces may be created and these forces need to be addressed by the appropriate muscles to avoid pain and strain, now or later.

For those who have been told that they have flat feet and require a particular type of supportive shoe or an orthotic in the shoe, I find the recommendation illogical. The arch of the foot is made up of a series of bones that are supported and maintained by muscles. Bones are innate and can't do anything on their own. Only when they are maintained in the proper position and alignment can they offer support, which is created by muscles. A widespread misunderstanding about the arch is that it is only supported by muscles in the foot, when, in fact, it is also controlled by the hip muscle, the gluteus medius.

Here's how it works: When you are single-leg standing, as with walking, the gluteus medius muscle is contracting to help keep your pelvis level, which gives you balance. If it is weak, the side of the pelvis opposite from the one you are standing on will have a tendency to drop. This will make you move from weight bearing in the middle of the foot to the inside of the foot, causing an excessive force through the arch. The two primary muscles that support the arch are the anterior and posterior tibialis muscles. With the excessive force applied to the arch, these muscles will take the load and they strain. Once strained, the arch fails and falls. So if you want to regain support of the arch, the key is to strengthen the gluteus medius muscle and the anterior and posterior tibialis muscles. The exercises that need to be performed are hip abduction, dorsiflexion, and inversion. (See pp. 196, 195, and 199 for instructions.)

A more supportive shoe or orthotic will create the support that muscles should be performing. This means the muscles not being used will weaken further, diminishing their ability to support the arch and, in effect, making your problem worse.

If you have pain at the underside of the foot, you most likely have a case of plantar fasciitis. The plantar fascia is a thick connective band that attaches from the balls of the feet to the heel. It is designed to help support the underside of the foot, including the arch. When the support of the arch is lost and the foot is flattened, the distance between the ball of the foot and the heel is increased. This puts stress on the plantar fascia and can irritate it, most often leading to pain at its attachment to the heel, but which can run along the underside of the foot. Resupporting the arch is the key to resolving this situation. This is achieved by strengthening the gluteus medius muscle and anterior and posterior tibialis muscles. The exercises to be performed are hip abduction, dorsiflexion, and inversion. (See pp. 196, 195, and 199 for instructions.)

In terms of shoes, whether they are lace-up, Velcro, or have some other form of fastening, as long as they have a nice supportive sole, that's really all you can ask of them. Your shoe style is your prerogative and should not be something determined by how much it plays into your health. If you are muscularly well conditioned, external elements will play a much less central role in the well-being of your body.

There have been times when my family decided to do some type of sightseeing activity spontaneously, which has involved extensive standing, negotiating difficult terrain or slippery surfaces, and all types of challenging circumstances to deal with. When the activities are on the spur of the moment, I am not always given the opportunity to have the best footwear for the journey. I have been challenged by wearing flip-flops or other unstable shoes, but because I am fit, I have been able to get through these types of activities without experiencing pain or limiting my enjoyment of the activity. You will always find yourself in situations where you are not prepared with the right clothes or the right equipment. But your health and fitness go with you wherever you are and will allow you to overcome any deficits that may present themselves from not being perfectly prepared.

As a general rule, sneakers are the most comfortable and supportive shoes that exist. They are made in so many different ways and for so many different purposes. Due to the fact that I am treating people throughout the course of the day, I am often standing. My wife found a sneaker with a marshmallow type of heel. It is very supportive and yet very lightweight. This means I am carrying less weight on my feet while standing, walking, kneeling, or any other activity I need to perform during the day. I like these and they feel good, so that works for me. I think the right sneaker for a person is up to them and simply depends on the type of activity they plan on performing. Comfort, in my mind, is the overriding sentiment that should determine a good sneaker.

I have been frequently asked whether I prefer regular sneakers or high-tops. Again, this really relates to the type of activity you are participating in. If the activity is very strenuous and sudden movement is a component, then increased ankle support may work for you. While the high-top sneaker can't prevent ankle sprains from happening, if there's risk of being stepped on or injured, they can certainly diminish the severity of damage. When I lift weights, I do like the feeling of a high-top supporting my ankle. It may be no more than a psychological comfort, but if it helps me lift better, I'm okay with that. All of that being said, remember, no sneaker can match the ankle or arch support created by strong and balanced muscles.

RUNNERS TAKE NOTE

There are many people out there who love to run. It allows you to look within yourself, to challenge what you can take. Most people have heard of runner's high. There is nothing like an adrenaline rush to put things in perspective and allow you to feel confident that things will work out just as you hope.

Unfortunately, a lot of people don't run with the proper technique and end up with pain in a variety of areas. Running, like any other activity, utilizes groups of muscles. All the muscles involved in performing the activity must be strong and balanced. That means if 10 muscles are required to perform an activity, 10 muscles must be strong and balanced to their opposing muscles. If only nine muscles are strong and balanced and one is weak, the nine muscles will have to take on the extra load of the weak muscle.

By now you know that muscles are not designed to take on any more than their assigned load, which means it is just a question of time before they break down and create unwanted symptoms. Your body and your mind want you to be happy, and if running makes you happy, your body and mind will decide you should continue running by finding a way to compensate for your imbalances. The variations in how you run may be so small that you don't even realize you have modified how you run, but those modifications to muscle function can accumulate to the point where you soon find running too painful to pursue. At this point, some doctors might tell you to simply stop running. But there is no earthly reason why you should stop doing something you love. My advice, instead, is to keep your muscles strong to prevent them from needing to compensate or modify movement. Isolated strength training will allow you to run with proper technique and without symptom.

Runners most typically develop pain at the lower back region, hip region, gluteal region, groin region, knee region, calf and shin region, ankle region, and feet. In all the cases I have treated, I have been able to find some muscle weakness or imbalance responsible for the cause of the symptoms. And after just a couple of weeks of strengthening, these patients were able to return to running with greater ease and increased enjoyment in the activity.

The first muscle that must be addressed for any runner to even have a remote chance of being able to run successfully without symptom is the gluteus medius muscle.

Fig. 6-1. Gluteus medius muscle

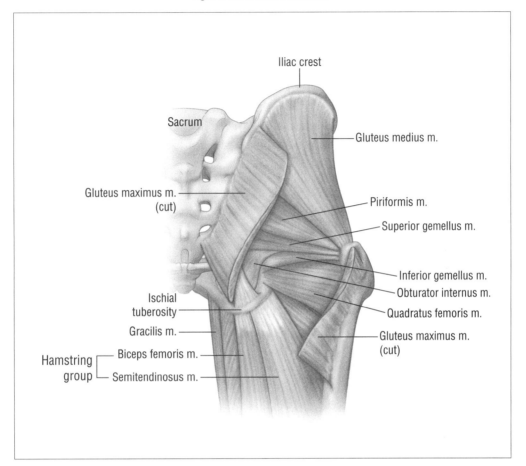

As you know, this is the muscle that sits just above the hip joint on the side of the pelvis, responsible for stability and balance, especially when standing on one leg. What makes running a little more challenging is the fact that at any one time, both legs may actually be off the ground. When the foot is placed down on the ground, the force the body must absorb is three and a half times your body weight, which occurs thousands of times every time you take a run. The gluteus medius acts as a shock absorber. When the foot is lifted off the ground, the weight of the leg pulls down on the attachment at the hip joint. The gluteus medius muscle contracts and controls this force until the foot is placed on the ground. In a sense, it allows the foot to be placed on the ground with a controlled force versus having a sudden force created when the body weight comes crashing down on the leg. To strengthen the gluteus medius muscle, perform the hip abduction exercise.

When looking at an elite runner while they are running, you will often see their ear is directly over their hip, meaning that their torso is perfectly upright. This is critical for maximizing energy and muscle output because when the torso is perfectly upright, the skeleton is in the perfect position to offset the force of gravity pushing down on the torso, where the weight of the torso is controlled by the skeleton and not the muscles. However, when most runners run, they are to some degree hip-flexed forward.

Fig. 6-2a. Normal posture   **Fig. 6-2b. Posture with hip flexed forward**

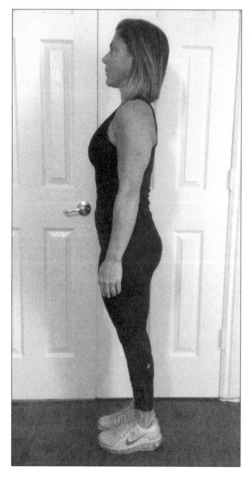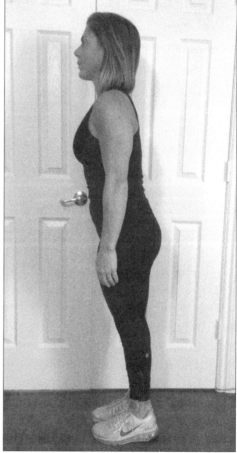

In effect, they are performing a controlled fall forward. For most people, this hip-flexed position means that the skeleton cannot support the torso, and therefore it must be supported by the lower back muscles. This can lead to strain and pain at the lower back.

If this is such as bad position, why can you find most runners doing it? The answer lies in the muscle imbalance that develops with activities like running. Since running is performed while moving forward, the muscles in the front of the pelvis and thigh, particularly the hip flexors and quads, must work hard to create the running motion. Since they are used more heavily than their opposing counterparts, the gluteus maximus and hamstrings, they will have a tendency to shorten. Because the hip flexors attach to the lumbar spine and the quads attach to the front of the pelvis, the torso is drawn forward into a hip-flexed position when they shorten. This means that an excessive load is created and the muscles of the lower back take the brunt of the load. For some people, the hip flexors can shorten enough and create the feeling that the back is being pulled into the stomach and can go into spasm, creating severe centralized lower back pain.

If this happens to you, your natural response might be to consider giving up running. Certainly, if you seek medical assistance and any structural variation is identified, such as a herniated disc, stenosis, or pinched nerve, this is the advice you will be given. But this does not have to be your destiny. The key to resolving this issue is to strengthen the opposing muscles to the hip flexors and quads, namely the gluteus maximus and hamstrings. To strengthen these muscles, you should perform the hamstring curl, hip extension, and straight leg deadlifts. To sustain the length of the hip flexors and quads while you are balancing out the opposing muscles, perform the hip flexor and quad stretches. (See pp. 196, 198, 204, 206, and 208 for instructions.)

Because of the load the gluteus medius plays in running, a few different muscles can be affected and lead to symptoms in different locations. The piriformis is a muscle that is located in the gluteal region. It sits next to the gluteus medius muscle. If the gluteus medius muscle strains, the piriformis will try to compensate and assist. Because it is not in the optimal position to provide stability and balance, it will strain and lead to pain at the gluteal region. This can be avoided by strengthening the gluteus medius and the muscles that work in conjunction with it, the hamstrings and gluteus maximus. The exercises to be performed are hip abduction, hip extension, hamstring curl, and straight leg deadlifts. (See pp. 196, 198, and 204 for instructions.)

If the piriformis strains significantly enough, it can thicken and impinge on the sciatic nerve, causing sciatic symptoms to run from the gluteal region down the leg to the foot. To resolve this situation, strengthen the gluteus medius, quads, gluteus maximus, and anterior tibialis. The exercises to be performed include hip abduction, knee extension, hip extension, and dorsiflexion. Once the symptoms no longer run down the leg and are just focused in the gluteal region, perform hip abduction, hip extension, hamstring curl, and straight leg deadlifts. (See pp. 196, 199, 198, and 195, and then 196, 198, and 204 for instructions.)

Another common pain associated with running is knee pain. It is often thought to be the result of osteoarthritis caused by the pounding and increased forces from running. However, in my experience, the cause in most cases has been a muscle imbalance between the quads (front thigh) and hamstrings (posterior thigh). The quads are heavily involved in the motion of running. Combine this with a hip-flexed posture while performing running, and you are putting an excessive load on the quads. This can cause them to shorten more than usual. Since the quads are connected to the kneecap via the quad tendon, the shortened quads can create an excessive upward force on the kneecap. This will cause the kneecap to be compressed in the knee joint when bending and straightening the knee, creating pain at the knee joint. Resolution of this issue comes from stretching the quads and strengthening the hamstrings and gluteus maximus. The exercises to be performed are the quad stretch, hamstring curl, hip extension, and straight leg deadlifts. (See pp. 208, 196, 198, and 204 for instructions.)

Another common cause of knee pain goes back to that strained gluteus medius muscle. If it strains another muscle called the tensor fascia lata, the ITB band, can try to compensate and strain. This causes the ITB to become shortened. Since it is attached to the outside of the kneecap, it can pull the kneecap laterally, causing it to impact the border of the knee joint and elicit pain. If you find it difficult to place the ankle of the leg with the painful knee on top of the knee of the unaffected leg, a shortened ITB is likely at fault. To resolve this issue, strengthen the gluteus medius, quads, gluteus maximus, and anterior tibialis. The exercises to be performed are the ITB stretch, hip abduction, knee extension, hip extension, and dorsiflexion. (See pp. 207, 196, 199, 198, and 195 for instructions.)

Some people might have pain in the groin region associated with running. This again relates to a strained gluteus medius muscle. If this muscle strains, it becomes hard to keep the pelvis level while standing on one leg. This will cause the pelvis to tilt down on the opposite side you are standing on, causing the muscles at the inside of the leg you are standing on to become shortened. Once shortened, the muscles lose their ability to create their maximal force and can strain. In this case, the muscle in question is the sartorius. Pain will come from the outer portion of the front of the pelvis into the groin region and reach down to the inner knee. Resolution occurs by strengthening the gluteus medius, gluteus maximus, and quads, and lengthening the sartorius muscle through the hip abduction, hip extension, knee extension, and sartorius exercises. (See pp. 196, 198, 199, and 201 for instructions.)

Many runners suffer from "shin splints," which are associated with the irritation of the muscle called the anterior tibialis. These muscles run along the lateral aspect of the lower leg bone called the tibia.

Fig. 6-3. Anterior tibialis

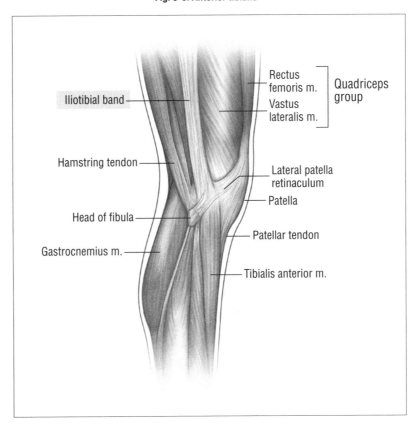

The forward posture or hip-flexed position that people find themselves running in will cause the body mass to lean in front of the hips, creating a load that has to be moved forward. The anterior tibialis muscles are responsible for picking the foot up before it swings forward to make the next step. With this load in the way, it is forcing the anterior tibialis muscles to have to work harder than they should. As a result, they strain and create pain at the lateral aspect of the front of the shin. When people have these symptoms, a common assumption is that something is wrong with the running sneaker. However, when people correct the excess stress on the anterior tibialis, the symptoms can be resolved. Resolution requires strengthening the gluteus maximus, gluteus medius, hamstrings, and anterior tibiails. The exercises to be performed are hip abduction, hip extension, hamstring curl, straight leg deadlifts, and dorsiflexion. (See pp. 196, 198, 204, and 195 for instructions.)

The same improper running technique may apply severely increased pressure at the balls of the feet. The excessive load applied to the balls of the feet can put more stress on the plantar fascia. As mentioned earlier, the plantar fascia is a thick connective tissue band that runs from the balls of the feet to the heel. If an excessive load is applied to the balls of the feet, the balls of the feet may separate or spread from the heel, causing undo stress to the plantar fascia and eliciting pain at the underside of the foot or at its attachment at the heel. To resolve this issue, you need to strengthen the gluteus maximus, gluteus medius, hamstrings, and anterior and posterior tibialis muscles. The exercises to be performed include hip extension, hip abduction, hamstring curl, straight leg deadlifts, dorsiflexion, and inversion. (See pp. 198, 196, 204, 195, and 199 for instructions.)

I have just presented multiple locations where pain might be elicited through running. In most cases, improper technique or the lack of muscle strength or balance is the culprit. However, by performing the proper exercises, the cause of the symptoms can be resolved and you can continue to run.

THE TRUTH ABOUT WALKING

You may have noticed that I have a real beef with the medical establishment over the pervasive and thoughtless prescription of walking. Even if you have pain when walking, you will most likely be told that you must keep walking. I have had patients who had hip or knee replacements and even back fusions, and all were told they needed to walk in order for their function to return. The reality in most of these cases was that their function did not return, and they ended up requiring assistive devices while continuing to have the pain they were experiencing before the surgery was performed.

To promote walking as the catchall answer to exercise is incredibly short-sighted. Unless they are engaged in an appropriate strength-training program, most people have weakness or imbalance of muscle. Telling these people to take regular walks is truly setting them up to develop symptoms and lose mobility. All activities require groups of muscles for performance. In order for the activities to be performed in a way that does not lead to symptoms and dysfunction, a person must begin by performing a targeted strength-training program. Once the muscles are strong and balanced, any activity can be performed safely and effectively.

In terms of cardiovascular exercise, walking does have its merits. But strength training is also cardiovascular. When strength training, muscle contraction causes lactic acid to be developed, which can result in the pH of the blood becoming acidic. The body doesn't want this to happen, so the heart sends increased blood flow to the muscles to bring the lactic acid to the liver for removal. It does so by pumping faster and harder. This creates a mechanism to strengthen the heart in the same light that walking, swimming or other "cardiovascular" exercises do. Anybody who has performed even the most rudimentary strength training would acknowledge that their heart pumps harder while doing the exercises.

Another problem with walking is that you don't use your arms. Walking is not going to help strengthen your arms for gardening or putting away dishes or performing other activities that depend on the arms. Even if you were to pump your arms while walking, it will not make them stronger. The only way to make muscles stronger is by adapting them to greater and greater resistance, which is the core principle of performing Yass Method exercises.

TRAVELING WITHOUT PAIN

Many people travel for enjoyment or are required to travel as part of their jobs. This can be very hazardous if you are not prepared for the loads that can be created. Just think about the moment when you reach the ticket counter and you are asked to put your bag up on the scale to see if it meets the weight requirement, which happens to be 50 pounds. You may not be appropriately conditioned to use your shoulder/shoulder blade and arm muscles, so you try to lean back a little to kick in the lower back muscles and *bam*—you just pulled your back out, which will make this trip difficult.

How about this scenario: You get on the plane and now it is time for you to put your carry-on in the overhead storage. You packed that bag pretty heavily with all the things you are going to need on the plane ride. You may not have conditioned yourself properly, and when you lift the bag over your head, you feel a pop at your shoulder and realize that you just strained your rotator cuff. For the rest of that trip, you better not plan on using that arm for much of anything.

Or perhaps you are taking a transcontinental flight, which could last for hours. You are stuck in that tight seat and you don't want to bother anybody to stand up and walk around the cabin, so you sit as long as you can and suddenly, your hip flexors go into spasm, creating massive back pain centered at the lumbar spine.

Then, of course, there is that last airport battle at the luggage carousel. You see your piece of luggage, which just squeaked under the 50-pound limit. It's coming at you and you have to jockey into place among everybody else trying to corral their bags. As it is moving, you find a way to stand it up enough to get a hold with one hand and then suddenly with all your might you have to lift this load over the lip of the carousel, which feels like it is two feet high but is really only about three or four inches. You take all that load on one side of the body and try to lower it to the ground and a shooting, stabbing pain develops in the gluteal region. You are finding it hard to stand up and have to sit down.

All of these opportunities for disaster present themselves and you haven't even left the airport. Now think about when you get to the rental car and you have to lift those bags into the trunk. And when you get to the hotel and reach your room, you are given what in my mind is one of the most bizarre of assistive devices—the fold-out luggage holder. It weighs about two pounds, seems to be made of balsa wood, and is held together with a couple of pieces of plastic straps, and you are supposed to lift your almost 50-pound bag onto this thing while it remains perfectly stationary?

Is it any wonder that most people think the actual traveling is the hardest part of any trip? And I agree 100 percent. So what should you do about these circumstances, and how can you avoid them? The answer remains the same—condition yourself for the forces involved in the activity. With traveling, there are upper body demands, back demands, and lower body demands, which I will present to you separately.

The Upper Body

Let's face the facts: you are going to have to carry a lot of heavy stuff. Sometimes lifting it from the floor to below waist height, and sometimes overhead. The key is that the support of the arms and anything that is lifted should be addressed by the muscles of the shoulder and shoulder blade. Even if you lift an object by bending the elbow and using the bicep muscle of the front upper arm, the ability of the bicep to work is only as effective as the shoulder blade held against the rib cage because the bicep actually is attached to the shoulder blade at its top.

The shoulder joint is the attachment of the upper arm bone into the end of the shoulder blade. The shoulder blade must be secured to the rib cage for normal arm function to occur.

Fig. 6-4. Shoulder joint

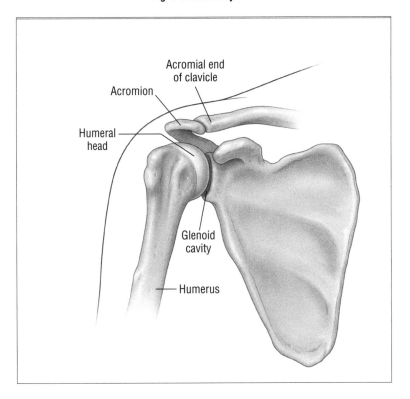

There is no joint capsule or ligament that performs this function. The two most important muscle groups responsible for normal shoulder and shoulder blade function are the mid-traps/rhomboids (interscapular muscles) and the lower trapezius. The interscapular muscles attach the shoulder blade to the spine. They keep the optimal distance between the spine and shoulder blades, so every muscle that attaches from the spine to the shoulder blades is maintained at its optimal length and creates its optimal force. For many people, their pecs (chest muscles), which oppose the interscapular (between the shoulder blades) muscles, get much stronger and can pull the shoulders forward, causing the shoulder blades to move away from the spine. This can lead to muscle failure and pain.

The lower trapezius, in my mind, is the hidden gem of muscles associated with shoulder and shoulder blade function. This muscle attaches to the shoulder blade and runs down to the lower thoracic spine. It is responsible for pulling the shoulder blade down the spine as the shoulder is lifted. This helps the muscles that are moving the arm bone in the shoulder joint as the arm is lifted. If this muscle is weak, other muscles involved in shoulder function can strain and emit pain.

The rotator cuff is a group of muscles that wraps around the head of the upper arm bone as it attaches into the shoulder joint. It plays a critical role in keeping the head of the upper arm bone from rising into the top portion of the shoulder joint when the arm is lifted.

The posterior deltoid is an important muscle in that it has to balance the force of the anterior deltoid, which sits at the front of the shoulder, and has a tendency to pull the head of the upper arm bone forward in the shoulder joint. This can lead to misalignment in the shoulder, creating pain. The posterior deltoid needs to be strengthened to equal the force of the anterior deltoid.

Finally, the portion of the tricep (posterior upper arm) muscle that attaches to the back of the shoulder joint needs to be strengthened to prevent the bicep, which sits in front of the upper arm and attaches to the shoulder joint as well, from pulling the head of the upper arm bone forward, which can lead to misalignment and pain.

As you can see, a lot of muscles are involved in securing the shoulder blade to the rib cage, as well as supporting the normal function of the shoulder joint. The shoulder joint's function is only as successful as the muscles involved in stabilizing and moving the shoulder blade. This is the area where the arm will get its ability to support anything that is held or moved, including the arm.

To combat the forces involved in traveling, strengthen the interscapular muscles, lower trapezius, rotator cuff, posterior deltoid, and triceps. The exercises to be performed are lat pulldown with neutral bar, lower trap, external rotation, posterior deltoids, and tricep extension. (See pp. 190, 188, 191, and 193 for instructions.)

Another point to note is the relationship between the shoulder/shoulder blade muscles and the neck. When people are getting pain at the neck/upper trap region, they have been programmed to believe it is associated with the cervical spine. The reality is that the cervical spine is connected to the shoulder/shoulder blade region. The upper trap area actually contains two big muscle groups, the upper trapezius and the levator scapulae. As mentioned, the name *levator scapulae* actually means "raise the shoulder blade," referring to the fact that although this muscle attaches at the top at the upper cervical spine, it is also attached to the shoulder blade and plays a major role in shoulder function.

When you sit for a prolonged period of time, such as on a flight, an altered posture associated with an imbalance of shoulder-based muscles can develop and cause neck pain. There is a tendency for the pecs (chest), anterior deltoids (shoulders), and biceps to become much stronger than the muscles between the shoulder blades, posterior deltoids, and triceps. This will cause the shoulders to be drawn forward, and a hunching in the upper back will develop. This posture causes the shoulder blades to move farther away from the spine. The muscles that support the head attach from the shoulder blades to the upper cervical spine, causing these muscles to become overstretched and lose their ability to create force. Slowly the head will lean farther forward, which is called forward head posture. Optimal posture would allow the back of the head to touch the seat as well and the head to be supported on the seat. This is not possible with improper posture, which creates a load that must be taken by the muscles that support the head. Over time, these straining muscles will create neck, upper back, or mid-back pain.

One short-term solution is to purchase a neck support. The doughnut-shaped pillows help to fill the gap between the back of the head and upper back, allowing your head to be supported when seated, even if it is slightly forward. Another way of addressing this issue is to recline your seat back. Most planes allow the seat to be reclined at least a little bit. Once the seat is angled back, gravity will move the head back and support it on the seat back. This can still be slightly uncomfortable, because if the forward head posture is severe enough, you will feel like your head has to point up in order to rest on the seat back. If you are using assistive devices, the combination of the neck support and reclined seat back would help to address this issue best. The next short-term mechanism that can be used is to stretch the pec muscles. This can be done to lengthen the pecs, which are the primary shortened muscles causing the hunched upper back position. By stretching your pecs, you can move the back of your head closer in line with your upper back and more easily rest your head on the seat back.

The long-term means to address this issue is to resolve the muscle imbalance between the pecs, anterior deltoids, and biceps versus the muscles between the shoulder blades, posterior deltoids, and triceps. This will correct the altered posture so that the back of the head is directly in line with the upper back. When sitting, both will touch the seat back and allow the head to be supported without difficulty, preventing overuse of muscle and pain. The muscles to be strengthened include the interscapular muscles (muscles between the shoulder blades), posterior deltoids, lower trapezius, rotator cuff, and triceps. The exercises to be performed include the lat pulldown with neutral bar, posterior deltoids, lower trap, external rotation, and tricep extension. (See pp. 190, 191, 188, and 193 for instructions.)

Just remember that the muscles involved in shoulder function attach to the spine all the way from the upper cervical spine down to the lower thoracic spine near the bottom of the rib cage. Any pain that is being experienced during sitting is most often associated with this muscle imbalance and can be resolved with this exercise regimen.

The Back

The lower back is an area that can be heavily affected by the forces associated with travel. Clearly, when wheeling suitcases around behind you, a load is developed at the lower back that must be taken by the lower back muscles. Lifting luggage from the floor to waist height or overhead will place major demands on the muscles of the lower back. But the act that can create the most peril for the lower back is where you appear to be doing almost nothing: sitting.

As part of the Yass Method, I reframe the thinking about how muscles are used and the possible causes of muscle strain and pain. Most people perceive tasks or actions as requiring movement. I want to change that concept. I want actions or tasks to include any activity that requires a change in position leading muscles to be maintained at altered lengths for any period of time. This would then include sitting. The reason why so many people have found sitting to be a major cause of lower back pain is because the muscles that attach from the hip joint to the lumbar spine, namely the hip flexors, change their length so dramatically when moving from a standing to a seated position. The hip flexors are at their optimal length when standing upright. This is called the neutral position of the hip joint, when the thigh is positioned directly under the torso. Now think about what happens when you sit and the angle between the torso and thigh. The angle becomes more acute, which is to say that the thigh moves closer to the torso. The angle between the torso and thigh becomes roughly 90 degrees, half of what it is when standing. This more acute angle allows the hip flexors to shorten substantially.

Fig. 6-5a. Angle between torso and thigh while standing

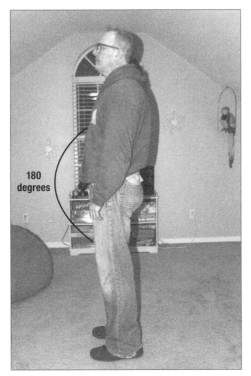

Fig. 6-5b. Angle between torso and thigh while sitting

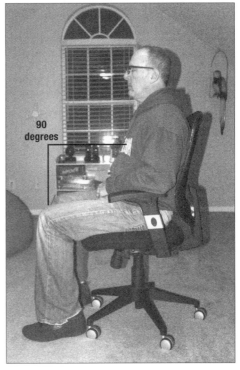

The hip flexors can shorten excessively if there is no opposing force from the gluteus maximus, the muscle that primarily opposes the hip flexors. Your back will feel like it is being pulled into your stomach. The attachment of the hip flexors to the lumbar spine will cause your lower back to arch. The hip flexors can even go into spasm, creating intense pain at the lower back region centralized near the spine. This is the primary reason people have lower back pain when sitting on an airplane for long periods of time. For some, it doesn't need to be long at all before the pain begins.

A couple of short-term and long-term options can be implemented to address this issue. One short-term option is getting up intermittently during the flight to allow the hip flexors to return to their normal length at standing, which can inhibit them from shortening further and eliciting pain. Another option is to find a place, possibly in the aisle or in the back of the plane, to perform a hip flexor stretch. This is basically kneeling with one knee stretched. It will provide short-term elongation of the hip flexors that will help diminish the lower back pain. A long-term solution is to strengthen the gluteus maximus and hamstring muscles. These are hip extensor muscles that oppose the hip flexors and, once strong enough, will prevent the hip flexors from ever getting short enough to strain and elicit pain, even with prolonged sitting. The exercises to be performed include the hip flexor stretch, hamstring curl, hip extension, and straight leg deadlifts. (See pp. 206, 196, 198, and 204 for instructions.)

The Lower Body

The biggest deterrent to being able sit for long periods of time on a plane during a flight is often knee pain, which relates to the issue of the hip flexors shortening. In this case, the muscle in question is the quadriceps (front thigh). The quadriceps run from the pelvis to the knee.

Fig. 6-6. Quadriceps

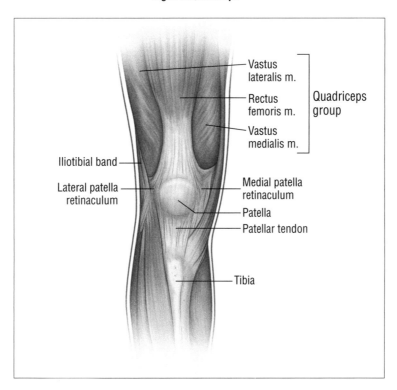

Vastus lateralis m. ⎤
Rectus femoris m. ⎬ Quadriceps group
Vastus medialis m. ⎦

Iliotibial band

Lateral patella retinaculum

Medial patella retinaculum

Patella

Patellar tendon

Tibia

While standing, the muscles are considered to be at their neutral length. When you sit, the knees bend to roughly 90 degrees. This can stretch the quads excessively. Since the muscle is attached to the knee joint via a tendon to the kneecap and then another tendon to the lower leg bone, or tibia, the shortening of the quads can create increased compression of the kneecap in the knee joint when the knee is bent. This increased compression can lead to irritation and pain at the knee joint. Sometimes you won't feel the pain until you try to stand up. But the reality is that the knee pain is due to an imbalance between the quads and hamstrings (posterior thigh), leading to the quads overshortening and the kneecap to be excessively compressed in the knee joint.

One short-term solution is getting up intermittently during the flight to prevent the kneecap from becoming excessively compressed in the knee joint. Another short-term solution is to stand up and find a convenient location to perform a quad stretch. For most, this can be performed in a standing position and will help to elongate the quads, preventing them from shortening and causing compression of the kneecap and knee joint. Finally, the long-term solution is to stretch the quads and strengthen the muscles that oppose them, which will help prevent them from shortening to the point where the kneecap will ever be compressed again. The muscles to be strengthened are the hamstrings and gluteus maximus. The exercises to be performed are the hamstring curl, hip extension, and straight leg deadlifts, along with a quad stretch. (See pp. 196, 198, 204, and 208 for instructions.)

Another big issue for people who might be seated for a long period of time on a flight is pain at the lateral thigh region. This is the result of a thickened connective tissue band called the iliotibial band, which attaches from the pelvis to the lateral knee.

Fig. 6-7. ITB

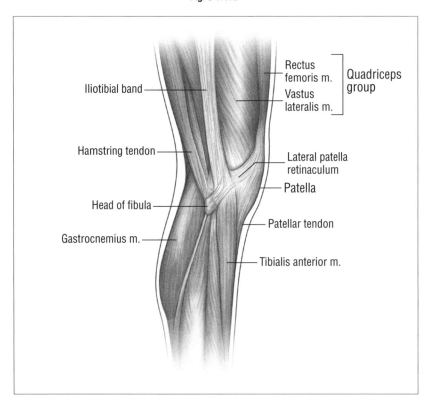

A small muscle at the top called the tensor fascia lata and the iliotibial band are involved in providing support and stability with weight-bearing activities, especially with single-leg standing. The primary muscle responsible for performing these tasks is the gluteus medius, which sits just above the hip joint on the side of the pelvis. When this muscle strains, other muscles try to compensate but can strain as well. Once strained, the ITB can become shortened. Since it attaches more toward the back of the knee, the ITB can also shorten if the knee is bent. If strained, the shortening will become excessive, and the ITB will elicit pain along the side of the thigh.

The first short-term mechanism to address this issue is to get up and stand or walk intermittently during the flight. This helps to keep the ITB at a more lengthened position, preventing it from shortening enough to elicit pain. Another short-term mechanism is to stretch the ITB. This is a stretch that can be performed while sitting. The problem is that the seats on a plane are pretty compact, so you might have to ask your neighbor if it is okay to perform the stretch. Finally, there is the long-term mechanism of strengthening the muscles responsible for the ITB straining and shortening. The muscles that would need to be strengthened include the gluteus medius, quads, and gluteus maximus. The exercises to be performed include hip abduction, knee extension, hip extension, and the ITB stretch. (See pp. 196, 199, 198, and 207 for instructions.)

DRIVEN TO PAIN

Commuting via car is a part of many people's day. Whether going to work or school or running errands for the home, driving is a way to get from point A to point B. If you live in a major city, traffic can be a part of your daily life. Even if you live in a rural area, the distance you might have to travel can keep you sitting in your car for long periods of time. The position that is maintained while sitting and driving can alter the lengths of muscles such that they can lead them to become strained and elicit pain. As you know by now, muscles can strain by being maintained at either very short or long lengths. One of the things I think people don't often realize is that although you are sitting when driving, you still have to support the weight of your torso, arms, and head. For most, the load is taken up by their muscles because they are not aware that positioning the seat back and the seat itself can help to absorb these forces or achieve the optimal position of the arms. Outstretched legs, especially the right leg, must be supported as well. There are tricks here in the following pages that can help minimize muscles of the neck, arms, back, and legs from overstretching or elongating to the point of eliciting pain.

The Neck

The best position for the seat back is where it is angled slightly behind upright; I would suggest about 10 degrees behind straight upright. Many people tend to have a rounded shoulder and forward head posture. So when they sit in a chair, even when their upper back is touching the chair, the back of their head is forward. This creates a load associated with supporting the head. This load has to be supported by muscles, namely the levator scapulae, which can strain and emit pain at the neck and upper trap region.

Fig. 6-8. Levator scapulae

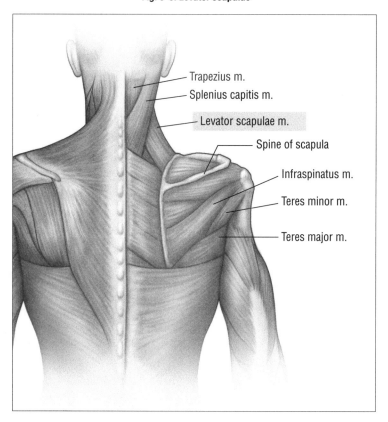

Trapezius m.
Splenius capitis m.
Levator scapulae m.
Spine of scapula
Infraspinatus m.
Teres minor m.
Teres major m.

If the seat is tilted back slightly, the body's center line will move behind the vertical position such that the body's weight, including the weight of the head, will be supported by the seat back, preventing the muscles from working too hard.

The long-term solution is to resolve the muscle imbalance between the pecs (chest), anterior deltoid, and biceps versus the muscles between the shoulder blades, posterior deltoid, and the triceps. The exercises to be performed are the lat pulldown with neutral bar, lower trap, external rotation, and tricep extension. (See pp. 190, 188, and 193 for instructions.)

The Arms

Most people never consider proper arm positioning to be of much importance and hold the wheel with the arm mostly extended. What they are missing is the fact that the arm is supported by the shoulder joint, meaning the shoulder blade, and thereby the torso. So while your torso may be supported by the seat back while driving, the shoulder blade and arm are actually not supported at all. This means something must be accepting this load, namely your muscles. The muscles involved in supporting the shoulder blades and arms are the levator scapulae, attached at the upper cervical spine, and the rhomboids and mid-traps, which connect to the thoracic spine between the shoulder blades. The lower trapezius muscles attach to the lower thoracic spine all the way down to the bottom of the rib cage. So technically, by sustaining the weight of your shoulder blades and arms freely when driving, you have the capacity to strain and elicit pain from muscles that run from the upper portion of the neck all the way down the mid-back to the level of the bottom of the rib cage.

The key thing to understand about weight is that the farther the weight moves away from the point where it is being supported, the greater the force that is created. For those lovers of physics, the equation for torque is applicable: force times distance. Why is torque so important to driving? Because it tells us that if you keep your arms fully extended while holding the steering wheel, you are moving the weight of the shoulder blades and arms farther away from the attachment to the torso, increasing the amount of load that must be supported by the muscles attaching from the shoulder blade to the spine. For a sustained period of time like a long drive, this is enough of a load to strain these muscles and cause pain.

Another pivotal muscle group involved in the support of the arm in the shoulder joint when the arm is held freely in front of the body is the rotator cuff. This muscle group keeps the arm bone in the shoulder joint and helps to maintain the proper distance of the head, or top, of the upper arm bone from the top of the shoulder joint. This space is needed for particular tendons to run freely without being impinged upon by the head of the upper arm bone. If the rotator cuff strains from having to support the weight of the arm bone in the shoulder joint when your arms are held out in front of you, it can lose its ability to sustain this space, causing pinching at the bicep tendon and eliciting pain at the front of the shoulder joint. I have treated innumerable patients who had rotator cuff strains leading to pinched bicep tendons in the shoulder joint. The onset of pain at the front of the shoulder when driving has been one of the key indicators of the cause of their distress.

The farther away your body is from the steering wheel, the higher your elbows have to rise. If your arms are almost fully extended to reach the steering wheel, your elbows will almost reach the height of your shoulders. This is the position where the greatest amount of force is required for the rotator cuff to keep the head, or top, of the upper arm bone from rising and pinching the bicep tendon. It is also the position where the weight of the shoulder blade and arm are farthest away from the torso, creating the greatest amount of force required from the muscles that attach the shoulder blade to the spine. This is clearly the worst possible position for the arms to be in while driving.

One possible short-term solution to prevent straining the muscles that support the arms while driving is to move the seat back to a point where the elbow is as close to below the shoulder as possible. For most, this is going to seem very different from the way you usually have your seat back. If your vehicle has armrests, by all means, use them to support your elbows. This takes the weight of your arms completely out of the equation and limits the chance for straining of the muscles that support the arms.

If all of this just feels too uncomfortable for you and you want to have your arms extended farther out to reach the steering wheel, then I would highly suggest intermittently alternating your hands while driving so that each arm will get an interval of supporting the weight of the arm as well as a chance to rest.

The long-term solution for driving optimally with your arms is to strengthen the muscles associated with support of the shoulder blades and the rotator cuff. The muscles to be strengthened include the muscles between the shoulder blades, posterior deltoids, rotator cuff, lower trapezius, and triceps. The exercises to be performed include lat pulldown with neutral bar, posterior deltoids, external rotation, lower trap, and tricep extension. (See pp. 190, 191, 188, and 193 for instructions.)

The Back

I am sure many people dread the idea of having to take a sustained drive because they get back pain. For some, just driving a short distance is enough to lead to severe pain. As with flying, the reason most drivers get back pain is shortened hip flexors. The hip flexors are the group of muscles that attach from the lumbar spine to the hip joint. If they become imbalanced to their counterparts, the gluteus maximus muscles (buttock), the hip flexors can shorten and create severe pain at the lower back, centralized to the lumbar spine. You will feel like your lower back has an excessive arch. A common recommendation is to get a lumbar support to fill the gap between the seat back and your lower back, but this just won't work. And there is a much better solution.

Maintaining your seat back at about 10 degrees behind straight upright will protect the neck and help support it so your muscles won't have to work so hard. This is actually a tremendously good position for the hip flexors as well. A straight upright position causes the angle between the torso and thigh to be roughly 90 degrees. The hip flexors are at their optimal length when the thigh is directly under the torso, such as when standing. If you create a 90-degree angle between the torso and thigh while sitting or driving with the seat back totally upright, the hip flexors will shorten excessively. If this position is maintained for a sustained period of time, the hip flexors will have a tendency to shorten further. Tone develops in the muscle, and the back will feel like it wants to be pulled into the stomach, creating the sensation of an increased arch. And if the right level of tension develops, the hip flexors will strain and elicit pain at the lower back.

By keeping the seat back about 10 degrees behind fully upright, the hip flexors will be kept at a more lengthened position, which can prevent that unhealthy muscle tone from developing. The torso will also have a tendency to lean back against the seat back in this position versus causing the lower back muscles to fully support the torso. This will reduce the tendency of the lower back muscles to make the hip flexors want to shorten further.

So setting your seat back to roughly 10 degrees behind fully upright is a good short-term solution for preventing lower back pain while driving. The long-term solution is to keep the hip flexors and quads at their optimal length by resolving any muscle imbalance between them and their opposing muscles, namely the gluteus maximus and hamstrings. The exercises to be performed include the hip extension, hamstring curl, and straight leg deadlifts, as well as hip flexor and quad stretches. (See pp. 198, 196, 204, 206, and 208 for instructions.)

Back pain does not have to be a part of driving. Understanding why the pain occurs and following the steps to prevent it will allow driving to become something you enjoy versus something you dread.

The Legs

The legs are similar to the arms in that the more the legs are extended, the greater the possibility becomes of muscles straining. The difference between the arms and legs is that the arms are basically free from support while the legs are supported by the bottom of the foot on the left leg or the heel of the foot on the right leg. A portion of the leg is also supported by the seat. A large portion of the back of the thigh rests on the seat, so the issue with the legs is less about straining from having to support the weight of the limb and more about how long the muscles stay in one position, which may cause the muscles to strain. When we look at the legs of a typical driver, the knees are usually fully extended. No muscle likes to be fully extended, especially for a sustained period of time. This can cause the muscle to want to recoil. The excessive tension that develops without the ability of the muscle to shorten creates enough force for strain.

The other issue relating to the legs is the fact that the right leg is typically balanced on the heel of the foot. This is a somewhat unstable position because the leg is creating a load that must be supported by the gluteus medius. The ITB and its attached muscle called the tensor fascia lata can assist the gluteus medius in providing support. If the gluteus medius is not strong enough, the tensor fascia lata and ITB might overcompensate and strain, leading to pain along the length of the ITB.

The short-term mechanism for preventing pain at the lateral aspect of the thigh or the back of the thigh is to maintain the knee bend at around a 30-degree angle from full extension. To accomplish this goal where no muscles are forced to sustain maximal lengths and thus no force of recoil is created, the seat must be moved forward or back in relationship to the position of the pedals.

The long-term mechanism for preventing leg pain while driving is to develop balance of the muscles of the front and back of the thighs, namely the hip flexors and quads versus the gluteus maximus and hamstrings. This will allow all the muscles to be able to hold at one length for sustained periods of time without feeling that they must recoil. The exercises to be performed include hip extension, hamstring curl, and straight leg deadlifts. To be able to sustain the legs, especially the right leg when balancing on the heel, strengthening of the gluteus medius is critical. The exercise to achieve this goal is hip abduction. (See pp. 198, 196, and 204 for instructions.)

TAKING A HIKE

Hiking is a wonderful recreational activity that can challenge the mind and the body. Depending on the severity of the terrain, it can be a mild workout or a hard workout. It is something that should not be taken lightly, even when it seems like it should be accomplished without much effort.

The nature of hiking typically implies that the terrain is not going to be level or smooth. Hiking can be performed on rocky terrains, muddy terrains, or other unstable terrains. As soon as you think *unstable*, I want you to immediately think about the muscles associated with providing stability and balance, namely the gluteus medius muscles. These muscles are the unsung heroes of the body. Your ability to sustain balance and stability lies almost exclusively with these muscles.

Let's say you are going to have to stand on the right leg for walking purposes or balance on a small surface. Here is how the gluteus medius works. If you look at your body, you will see that the majority of your body weight is to the left of the right leg. So if you were to take your left foot off the floor and stand just on the right foot, your body would fall to the left side. If you think of your right leg as the base of a teeter-totter, on the left side of the teeter-totter would be your body weight. Think of your weight as a force being pushed toward the ground. On the right side of the teeter-totter, something must create the equivalent force of your body weight to make the teeter-totter level. This is the gluteus medius muscle, which is attached to the outside of the pelvis and the hip joint. When you create a force toward the outside of the right leg that is equal to the force represented by your body weight, your pelvis will maintain a level position and you will balance on the right leg even with the left leg off the floor.

If we go back to the idea of hiking on unstable or uneven surfaces, you can imagine just how much more force will be required of the gluteus medius muscles to support you. If the gluteus medius muscles are not strong enough for this increased demand, they can strain and elicit pain just above the hip joint on the side of the pelvis. Or they can cause other muscles to try to compensate for the lack of ability to address the forces being created. This can cause the piriformis to strain and elicit pain at the gluteal region, the ITB to strain and elicit pain at the lateral aspect of the thigh and knee, the sartorius muscle to strain and elicit pain at the groin region down the inner knee, or the quadricep muscles to strain and elicit pain at the front thigh or knee. If you plan on hiking, you must prepare by strengthening the gluteus medius muscles through hip abduction. (See p. 196 for instructions.)

Since the terrain for hiking may involve inclines, make sure you are prepared for the increased loads involved. The muscles associated with addressing inclines are the quadricep muscles, which are at the front of the thighs. To strengthen them, perform knee extensions, lunges, or squats. I prefer lunges or squats because you are weight-bearing when performing these exercises, so there is greater stability created at the knee joint and less chance for injury.

When strengthening the quads, it is critical to recognize that these muscles are typically stronger than their opposing muscles, the hamstrings. It is always advisable to simultaneously strengthen the hamstrings when strengthening the quads, lest you exacerbate the muscle imbalance and cause the quads to shorten excessively, leading to strain or an excessive arching of the lower back. This can then strain the lower back muscles and lead to back pain or pull the kneecap into the knee joint excessively, leading to compression of the kneecap and pain at the knee joint. Maintaining balance of the quads and hamstrings prevents a whole host of problems from arising. To strengthen the hamstrings and the quads, perform hamstring curls and straight leg deadlifts. (See pp. 196 and 204 for instructions.)

To maximize the muscles of the legs working to help you hike, it is important that the torso be maintained over the hips so that it is supported by the skeleton, which requires no energy and in fact leads to energy efficiency. Less energy having to go to the support of the torso means more energy that can focus on moving you along. If the torso is maintained in a flexed position, a load is being created in front of the hip joint that has to be supported by some muscles. This is typically going to be picked up by the lower back muscles. If they are forced to overwork, they can strain and emit pain at the lower back. To sustain a position where the shoulders are maintained over the hips and the torso is held in an upright position, the muscles that must be strengthened are known as the hip extensors. These muscles attach from the thigh to the pelvis in the back of the body and create an upright posture and include the gluteus maximus and hamstrings. The exercises to be performed include hip extension, hamstring curl, and straight leg deadlifts. (See pp. 198, 196, and 204 for instructions.)

Due to the instability of the terrain you might encounter, ensuring that your ankle muscles are strong will prevent against ankle sprains and also create a strong foundation. If your ankles are strong and stable, everything on top of the ankles will be more stable and require less force due to better stability. The muscles most associated with creating stability at the ankles include the anterior and posterior tibialis. The exercises to be performed include dorsiflexion and inversion. (See pp. 195 and 199 for instructions.)

One small point about footwear can be made. Clearly, shoes with strong soles and good side support should be worn when hiking. But simply wearing these types of shoes will not prepare you to take on the increased forces associated with hiking. Just like any other activity, the force requirements of the activity must be met evenly by the force output of the muscles performing the activity to prevent strain and pain.

WHEN CLIMBING IS THE PROBLEM

I have treated many people who have said that they can stand or walk with no problem, but negotiating stairs is almost impossible. It might not even be pain that is limiting them. It might be that they simply cannot support themselves on one leg while moving their other foot to the next stair. When the pain is at the knee, the natural tendency is to seek medical care, where you are often told that you require a joint replacement. Let me explain why this is crazy. First of all, the X-ray is not capable of determining whether you are truly bone on bone, meaning that there is actually zero joint space. Even if there is just a slight space, a joint has the capacity to work perfectly. Secondly, range of motion is the determining factor as to whether someone is bone on bone. To check this, the joint must be moved through range of motion passively by another individual to see if full range of motion can be achieved. Pain is not a determining factor. The only factor is whether full range of motion can be achieved. If it can, there is no question— the joint cannot be bone on bone.

Negotiating stairs involves your body weight applying substantial force to the joint. If there is a muscular deficit, a misalignment of the joint surfaces can occur, leading to pain at the joint. This has absolutely nothing to do with the range of motion of the joint that is available. The failure to negotiate stairs is pretty much a clear indication of a muscular deficit. Let's take two separate cases, which have two different causes. The first is where knee pain is the inhibiting factor when negotiating stairs. The second case is where the ability to support one's self is in question, because the knees seem to buckle when trying to negotiate stairs.

In the case where knee pain is the primary factor preventing the person from negotiating stairs, pain associated with going up the stairs may have a different cause than pain experienced going down the stairs. When going up stairs, the knee doesn't have to bend more than 90 degrees. The quad (front thigh) muscle is contracted to extend the knee and raise you to the next stair. The two primary reasons for pain when going up stairs are that either the quads are too strong in relationship to the hamstrings or the quads have strained. In the first case, the quads have shortened and, due to the imbalance and the attachment of the quad to the kneecap via the quad tendon, an excessive upward force will be created on the kneecap. This upward force will cause the kneecap to be excessively compressed in the knee joint. When the quad is contracted to lift your body weight to the next stair, the excessive compression might lead to pain at the knee joint. The key to resolving this issue is to stretch the quads and strengthen the hamstrings to elongate the quads. The exercises to be performed include the quad stretch, hamstring curl, and straight leg deadlifts. (See pp. 208, 196, and 204 for instructions.)

With the second possibility, if the quad has strained, the kneecap will tend to glide more to the side of the knee joint. This means the kneecap can actually contact the lateral border of the knee joint. When your body weight is lifted by contracting the quad to go up the next step, the irritation of the kneecap contacting the lateral border of the knee joint can elicit knee pain and may create a cracking or snapping sensation. The key to resolving this issue is strengthening the quads so that they run through the knee joint properly. The exercises to be performed in this case are knee extension, squats, and hamstring and calf stretches. (See pp. 199, 202, 206, and 205 for instructions.)

In either case, balance will be a factor and therefore strengthening of the gluteus medius muscle is always advisable. To achieve this, perform hip abduction. (See p. 196 for instructions.)

In the case where going down stairs elicits knee pain, the cause is slightly different. When going down stairs, you are standing on one step and you have to bring your foot down to the next step below. This means that the knee joint of the leg you are standing on will have to go through more than 90 degrees of motion and instead undergo more like 115 degrees of motion. If your quads are shortened due to a muscle imbalance between the quads and hamstrings, the kneecap may compress into the knee joint with greater force than it should be. This means the more the knee is bent, the more compressed the kneecap becomes. With the amount of knee range of motion needed to go down stairs, the increased compression of the kneecap from a shortened quad can be enough to elicit pain at the knee, preventing you from being able to step down the staircase. Some people even go down steps sideways to compensate for this difficulty. To resolve this issue, perform quad stretches, hamstring curls, and straight leg deadlifts. Since we are talking about single-leg standing, I also recommend strengthening the gluteus medius for balance and stability through hip abduction. (See pp. 208, 196, 204, and 196 for instructions.)

Finally, I want to talk about a case where it seems like the knee joints are buckling in, preventing your ability to negotiate stairs. This is a very different circumstance than when the knees stay directly under the hips. When the knees seem to buckle in, even when there is pain at the knee joints, the cause is actually at the hips. I must say that it has surprised me to learn how many people have ended up in this circumstance. You can see this to a lesser degree when a person encounters difficulty in going from sitting to standing because the knee is not kept under the hip. When the knee caves in due to lack of gluteus medius muscle strength, the quads, which are trying to lift you, cannot create force. They can only pull off a rigid post when the thigh and lower leg bones are maintained under each other. Without the gluteus medius's contractile force pulling outward on the thigh to keep the knee joint under the hip joint, rising from a chair to a standing position is almost impossible. Now imagine raising your body the height of a step by pushing down on one leg to raise the other. If standing up from a chair is difficult with two legs, negotiating stairs with one leg at time would certainly feel almost impossible.

In this instance, the reason for the knees caving in is that only a small portion of the joint is in a position to support you, versus when the knee is directly under the hip. This is going to cause muscles to have to work much harder and can lead to strain and misalignment of the joint surfaces between the kneecap and the knee joint. Because the pain is at the knee joint, the person may naturally assume that the cause of the pain is the structure of the knee joint. With just a simple visit to a surgeon who is trained to identify structural variations of a joint, even when they are not causing pain, you have all the makings of an unnecessary joint replacement to add to your difficulties.

When I have been asked to diagnose the cause of a person's knee pain, patients have presented with buckled knees while they stood or walked, to the point where their knees were almost touching one another. I would ask the person if they realized just how buckled their knees were and, to my surprise, they said no. If I asked them to stand on one leg, the knee would collapse in with just trying to take one foot off the floor. It was appalling to think that other medical practitioners had convinced the person the problem was at the knee simply because the pain was being experienced there.

The presentation of the body's symptoms always tells the tale of what tissue is responsible for the symptoms experienced. When a person's knees buckle in, it is because the gluteus medius muscles (which sit above the hip joint and attach to the side of the pelvis) have strained severely and cannot keep the knee under the hip when standing. This is grossly obvious but rarely identified because the practitioner is not educated to evaluate the presentation of the body's symptoms.

To resolve the issue of the knees caving in while negotiating stairs, you should strengthen the gluteus medius. You should strengthen the quads as well, because these muscles raise or lower you as you move from step to step. For the quads to work correctly, the knee must be maintained under the hip joint. As such, when performing squats, it is important for the range of motion to keep the knee under the hip at all times. Strengthening of the gluteus maximus is also important, as it is a key hip extensor muscle and will help to keep the torso upright so the shoulders remain over the hips when negotiating stairs. The exercises to be performed are hip abduction, squats, and hip extension. (See pp. 196, 202, and 198 for instructions.)

This is a case where it might take a little longer to see the results of the strengthening to improve the ability to negotiate the stairs. Improvement will first be seen when raising and returning to a sitting position.

Just remember that the primary mechanical failure is the knee not being maintained under the hip to create a strong post for the quads to pull off to lift or lower you when negotiating the stairs. A combination of strengthening the gluteus medius along with a conscious attempt to keep the knee under the hip during the action will help you to regain your ability to negotiate stairs painlessly.

EXERCISES USED IN THIS CHAPTER

Fig. 6-9a. Beginning of hip abduction exercise

Fig. 6-9b. End of hip abduction exercise

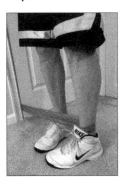
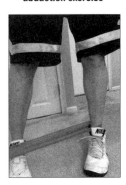

Fig. 6-9c. Beginning of hip abduction exercise

Fig. 6-9d. End of hip abduction exercise

Fig. 6-9e. Side view of hip abduction exercise

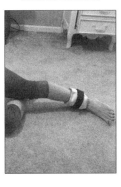
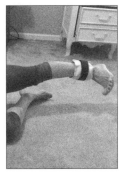
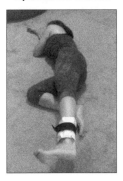

Fig. 6-10a. Beginning of hamstring curl

Fig. 6-10b. End of hamstring curl

Fig. 6-11a. Beginning of hip extension

Fig. 6-11b. End of hip extension

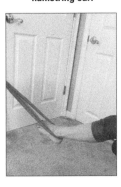
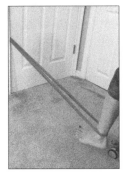
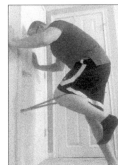
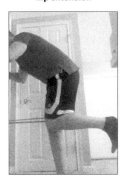

Fig. 6-12a. Beginning of straight leg deadlifts

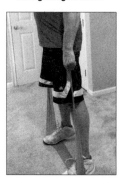

Fig. 6-12b. End of straight leg deadlifts

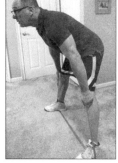

Fig. 6-13a. Beginning of dorsiflexion

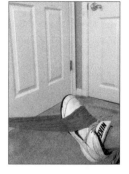

Fig. 6-13b. End of dorsiflexion

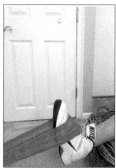

Fig. 6-14a. Beginning of inversion

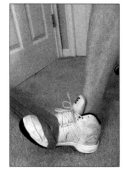

Fig. 6-14b. End of inversion

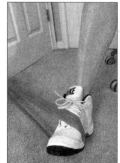

Fig. 6-15. Hip flexor stretch

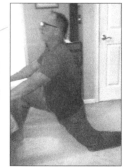

Fig. 6-16. Quad stretch

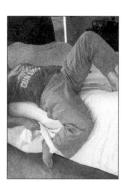

Fig. 6-17a. Beginning of knee extension

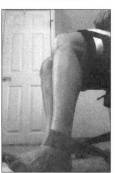

Fig. 6-17b. End of knee extension

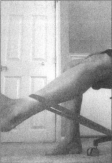

Fig. 6-18. ITB stretch

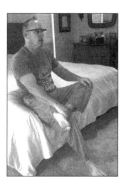

Fig. 6-19a. Beginning of sartorius exercise

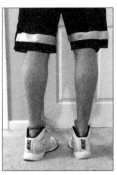

Fig. 6-19b. End of sartorius exercise

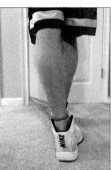

Fig. 6-20a. Beginning of lat pulldown

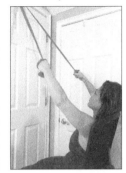

Fig. 6-20b. End of lat pulldown

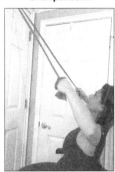

Fig. 6-21a. Beginning of posterior deltoids exercise

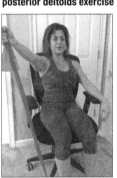

Fig. 6-21b. End of posterior deltoids exercise

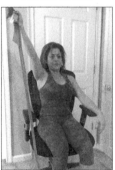

Fig. 6-22a. Beginning of lower trap exercise

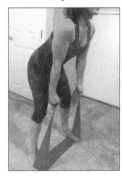

Fig. 6-22b. End of lower trap exercise

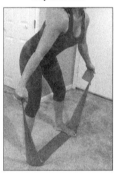

Fig. 6-23a. Beginning of external rotation

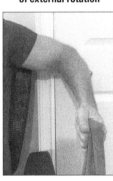

Fig. 6-23b. End of external rotation

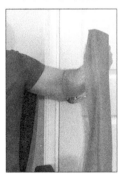

Fig. 6-24a. Beginning of tricep extension

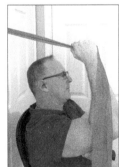

Fig. 6-24b. End of tricep extension

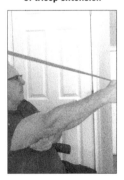

Fig. 6-25a. Beginning of squats

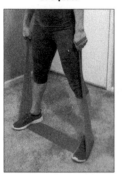

Fig. 6-25b. End of squats

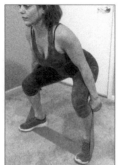

Fig. 6-26. Hamstring stretch

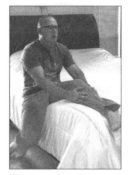

Fig. 6-27. Calf stretch

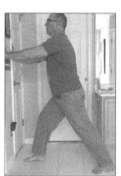

CHAPTER SEVEN

Special Situations and Aging

UNDERSTANDING YOUR PREDISPOSED CONDITIONS

Oftentimes people experiencing pain cannot recall a specific incident that initiated their pain or even pinpoint when the pain began. Of course, in the case of a car accident or a major fall, the cause is obvious and is associated with trauma. But for the vast majority of those I have treated, the original scenario is the one that most describe. How can it be that you can suffer from such levels of pain without being able to recall a specific event or time when the pain began? I think a deeper understanding of the cause of pain would show us just how little has to be done to stop it or, perhaps more importantly, prevent it from recurring.

The Yass Method is based on the theory that most people are suffering from chronic pain because they don't have enough strength in all their available muscles to perform daily activities. The core force that the muscles are working against is gravity, so some type of force is going to have to be exerted by muscles in any activity where you are not completely lying flat on the floor. Of course, your body weight, the strenuousness of the activity, and a variety of metabolic considerations—such as what you have eaten, how much you have slept, or how much you are stressed—will affect the amount each muscle is involved in creating its portion of the total force needed to perform the activity.

To tackle this from another angle, consider this: You have two legs and therefore it seems logical that one leg should take 50 percent of your body weight while the other leg should take the other 50 percent. But let's say you just dropped a heavy bag on the floor and need to pick it up. There are two ways you might achieve this goal. You might straddle the bag and bend down, bearing your weight equally on both legs, or maybe you bend and lift the bag to your side instead of between your legs. Without realizing it, you caused yourself to support 80 percent of your body weight on the leg nearest to the object being lifted. This one small variation could lead to strain now and possibly pain later.

Another point to consider is that the ability to achieve our goals leads to success. The body was designed with an ability to create complex movement without conscious thought. It makes demands of the muscles to complete tasks without verifying whether the muscles are capable of doing so. If a muscle strains, the body does not typically create conscious awareness of the strain. When the muscles used for simple daily activities such as standing, walking, or kneeling have to overwork, they strain and cause you to feel pain. But they still say to the body, *We can get the job done.* Knowing this about your body, it's up to you to decide how you do that job.

Why do we allow ourselves to be in pain? Why don't we have a daily checklist to see if the muscular system is still functioning properly? A simple examination to see where the ear, shoulder, and hip lie in relation to one another can help to determine if an imbalance is leading to a substantial enough change in posture such that it may cause symptoms to develop. With proper posture, the ear, shoulder, and hip will all be in alignment when looking at yourself from the side. Forward head and shoulder posture will give the appearance of having an excessive hunching at the upper back.

THE AGE OF YOUR PAIN

Countless people have been suffering with chronic pain for years. Many have been told the cause of the pain is structural, such as a herniated disc, arthritis, pinched nerve, stenosis, or meniscal tear. When the pain is unresolved after procedures and surgeries, it may feel as if things are getting worse simply because time is passing. This mind-set will often convince a person that surgery is the only option or that pain management is all that is left. There is a belief that the longer time passes with the pain persisting, the ability to resolve the pain decreases. This is where hopelessness and depression find their way into the mix.

Contrary to popular belief, if the cause of the symptoms is muscular, then time does not play much of a factor at all. Muscular causes can be resolved in just a few weeks or a couple of months, depending on the severity of the weakness of the muscles.

On innumerable occasions, I have treated people who have been experiencing pain for years. They have been told the cause is structural and have attempted every type of treatment available through the medical establishment. It is now 10 years down the road from when the pain began. Through some circumstance, the person finds out about me and the Yass Method. They seek treatment from me. I establish that the cause of their pain is muscular. I perform treatment to maximize the lengths of the muscles and improve their force output. We perform targeted progressive resistance exercises, and within just a couple of days the symptoms are resolved and full function returns. Full of emotion from a decade's worth of pain and frustration, the person says to me, "Wow, it took me ten years and one week to resolve my pain. How horrible is that?" I reply, "Actually, it only took you one week to resolve the cause of your pain."

It is important to understand that the duration of chronic pain is not necessarily an indication of how severely the tissue is deteriorating. For almost every person I have ever come in contact with, the time frame of chronic pain is merely an indication of the time spent identifying and treating the wrong tissue. Don't interpret the duration of chronic pain as meaning that you are moving further and further away from the opportunity to resolve the cause of the symptoms. In most cases, chronic pain is the result of misdiagnosed acute pain. So if the cause at the initial phase was muscular but was not identified properly, even if it is finally identified and treated years after the pain began, the cause can be resolved just as easily as when the symptoms first appeared.

Time can be a factor in resolving muscular deficits, but it is not due to muscles decaying over time. If one particular muscle is too weak, another will try to compensate, causing multiple muscles to strain. Eventually, life's activities will be performed by fewer and fewer healthy muscles. When I treat patients who have had pain for years or even decades, I typically see the most extreme alterations in how they perform their daily activities. People might be walking or standing with their knees touching one another for support or waddling with an extreme side bend to walk. They might be hip-flexed so far forward that it would only take the lightest pressure to make them fall forward. I'm often impressed by the body's ability to integrate muscles into activities they were never designed to be involved in.

The good news is that the age of your pain is not even remotely an indicator of how difficult it will be to resolve the true cause of your pain. For most, time has been just holding a place until the right mechanism to diagnose the true cause of pain can be identified. Once identified, the cause can typically be resolved in just days, weeks, or a couple of months. So please be optimistic. There is no reason for hopelessness. Look forward to a future of pain-free living and put the past where it belongs—behind you.

MUSCLE STRENGTH AND BALANCE

I have come in contact with so many people who have gone down the path from independent movement to being wheelchair-bound. In almost every case, I was able to help them reverse the path so they could return to independent movement again. The difference is not magical—it is simply understanding when balance is compromised due to a muscular deficit versus a neurological deficit. Guiding people back to independent movement has taught me to reject the notion that instability is an inevitable result of aging.

I have treated many people who have had balance issues, as they'd mentioned that they found themselves tripping a lot. Oftentimes, they would fall but were able to catch themselves before reaching the ground. If you are not a senior, it is usually called being clumsy. But if you are a senior, many consider it a balance deficit. This is an attitude clearly borne of age discrimination, which needs to be eliminated.

Let's discuss the two general aspects of balance: your awareness of where you are in space, and your ability to adapt to this if you become unstable. The ability to sense where you are in space comes primarily from a structure in your ears called the semicircular canals. This structure is designed to make up your point of reference from three planes: the forward to back, side to side, and horizontal. By referencing your position in space via these three planes, your brain determines how to be upright. If there is a deficit that affects this process, your ability to understand in what way you are upright is compromised and doing anything

174

other than lying flat will be difficult to achieve. Those who have had an ear infection affecting the semicircular canals can attest that doing anything other than lying down during this period is very difficult.

Most of the people I have treated who were told that their balance issue was due to a neurological deficit could, in fact, do anything they wanted other than perform weight-bearing activities.

Here is a simple test to see if your problem in performing weight-bearing activities is neurological in nature. Sit in a chair with no support from armrests or the seat back. Your torso should be completely free from support. If you can sit with no support, this implies that the neurological aspect of balance is intact. You are able to support the torso, which means that you still possess the ability to identify the upright position. So if you find that you are capable of supporting yourself while sitting, what is the problem when it comes to performing weight-bearing activities?

Let's say that you are standing up. Your neurological system is functioning properly and you start to notice that you are beginning to lean to one side. You can feel you are becoming unstable and the brain begins sending signals to muscles on the side you are leaning toward to contract and push you back toward the stable upright position. But what if these muscles are too weak to create the force necessary to stop you from leaning? And what happens if you lean so far to the side that your center of mass extends beyond the leg supporting you? You will fall. You will be told you have a "balance problem." You will be told you are too unstable and you require an assistive device.

But what is really the problem? Your muscles are too weak, plain and simple.

Your neurological system did its job. It sensed you were leaning to the side. It sent signals to your muscles to move you back to upright. But the muscles were too weak to respond, so you fell. This is not a case of balance; this is a case of muscle weakness. And this is the situation I have found in almost every person I have treated who was diagnosed with instability. Balance is not an independent element. It is a combination of two elements: neurological function and strength. As mentioned, for most people, the ability to sense where they are in space is generally intact. The problem is that the muscles typically associated with creating stability are not strong enough.

The two primary ways people fall are to the side or forward. The muscles that are involved in providing stability side to side are the gluteus medius. The muscles involved in preventing falling forward are the gluteus maximus and hamstrings.

The feeling of falling to the side stems from the fact that the pelvis is not kept level while standing or walking. This tilting of the pelvis will cause the torso to tilt to the same side, altering the center of body mass. This means more weight is being moved toward the side. The muscles of one leg are being asked to support this movement of weight, which is greater than the load the muscles were intended to take. This is why they fail to hold you up when you continue to tilt and finally fall toward that side.

The muscles responsible for keeping the pelvis level when weight-bearing and, more importantly, when single-leg standing are the gluteus medius muscles. Because of its attachment to the side of the pelvis, the gluteus medius is responsible for creating an equivalent output to balance your body weight on the leg you are standing on. When this happens, the pelvis is kept level and balance is secured. If the muscle is weaker and creates less force than the equivalent of your body weight, gravity wins the battle and you tilt to the opposite side, making you susceptible to falling. However, this lack of balance can easily be avoided and prevented by strengthening the gluteus medius muscle of the leg on the opposite side that you seem to fall toward.

Weakened gluteus medius muscles can also cause your feet to move closer together while standing or walking. Because the legs are maintained in a vertical position, the optimal position for the feet when standing or walking is directly under the hips. Since gravity is pushing down vertically, the skeleton has the ability to work directly against gravity to support you. This makes your body more efficient, creating less work for your muscles. But when your feet move in toward the midline with weak gluteus medius muscles, your base of support narrows. This makes it easier for your center of body mass to move outside your feet, making you more susceptible to falling to the side.

If instability has developed, the use of a cane can be an appropriate response in the short term. The cane should be placed on the side that you are falling toward to stop the momentum of the body from moving in that direction. But in addition to a cane, a progressive resistance exercise program should be implemented to strengthen the affected gluteus medius muscle along with any other muscles that may have weakened with it. By performing a progressive resistance exercise program, strength will develop in all the appropriate muscles so that the legs can support you fully and you can regain stability. The most typical muscles that tend to be weakened alongside the gluteus medius muscle are the gluteus maximus and hamstrings. The exercises used to strengthen these muscles are hip abduction, hip extension, hamstring curl, and straight leg deadlifts. (See pp. 196, 198, and 204 for instructions.)

Fig. 7-1a. Beginning of hip abduction exercise

Fig. 7-1b. End of hip abduction exercise

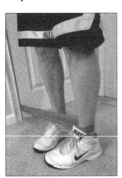
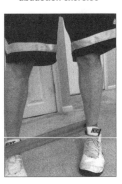

Fig. 7-1c. Beginning of hip abduction exercise

Fig. 7-1d. End of hip abduction exercise

Fig. 7-1e. Side view of hip abduction exercise

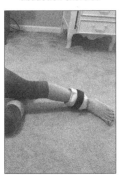
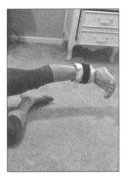
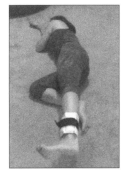

**Fig. 7-2a. Beginning
of hip extension**

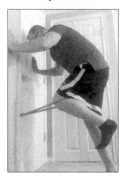

**Fig. 7-2b. End
of hip extension**

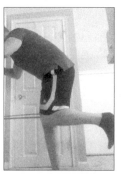

**Fig. 7-3a. Beginning
of hamstring curl**

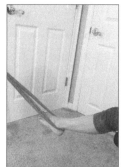

**Fig. 7-3b. End
of hamstring curl**

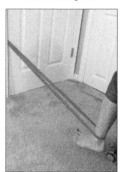

**Fig. 7-4a. Beginning of
straight leg deadlifts**

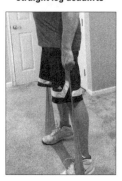

**Fig. 7-4b. End of straight
leg deadlifts**

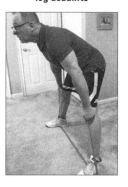

After you regain stability, you can return to normal function without a cane, walker, wheelchair, or other assistive device.

For those who have a tendency to fall forward when losing their balance, a muscle imbalance between the hip flexors and quadriceps versus the gluteus maximus and hamstrings is often the cause. The hip flexors and quads have a tendency to develop and become stronger than the gluteus maximus and hamstrings, which causes these muscles to become shortened. In shortening, they have a tendency to cause a person to sustain a hip-flexed posture. This causes the ear to be more in line with the mid-foot or toes when looking from a side view, versus having the ear over the ankle. This will create a load over the front of the ankle. If the gluteus maximus and hamstrings are weak, the individual will have difficulty slowing momentum from being developed in a forward motion. So when you walk, you might feel like you are performing a controlled fall forward. When standing, you might feel like your center of mass is moving in front of your toes. Either way, you will fall forward.

Other signs that the hip flexors and quads are shortened and leading to this forward center of mass are pain at the lower back or the knees when standing after sitting for a while, and a postural presentation of the ear being in line with the mid-foot or toes when looking at yourself from the side.

The way to resolve this issue is to stretch the quads and hip flexors and strengthen the gluteus maximus and hamstrings. The exercises to achieve this goal include the quad stretch, hip flexor stretch, hamstring curl, hip extension, and straight leg deadlifts. (See pp. 208, 206, 196, 198, and 204 for instructions.)

Fig. 7-5. Quad stretch   **Fig. 7-6. Hip flexor stretch**   **Fig. 7-7a. Beginning of hamstring curl**   **Fig. 7-7b. End of hamstring curl**

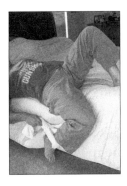 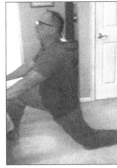 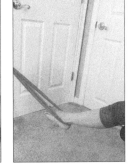 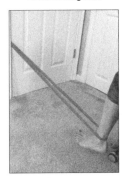

Fig. 7-8a. Beginning of hip extension   **Fig. 7-8b. End of hip extension**   **Fig. 7-9a. Beginning of straight leg deadlifts**   **Fig. 7-9b. End of straight leg deadlifts**

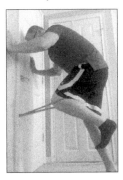 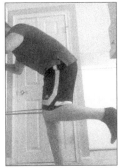 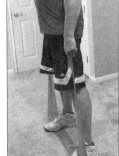 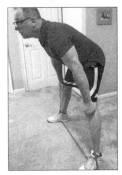

If you have a tendency to trip when walking, even if you don't necessarily fall, identify the foot that catches when you trip. Then stand on one foot using that leg and then single-leg stand on the opposite foot. Do this for a few seconds. If it feels about the same, then try to single-leg stand and bend the knee of the leg you are standing on three times. Determine which side it is harder to do this test with. I bet you will see that it is much harder to single-leg stand or single-leg squat on the leg opposite the foot that catches you when you trip. Just as with people who have a tendency to fall, essentially the same thing happens to the pelvis when the gluteus medius on one side is weak: the pelvis will tilt down on the opposite from the weak gluteus medius, decreasing the distance between the pelvis and the floor on one side, making less room for the foot to be swung through when stepping forward. This is why the foot catches and you trip. It's not clumsiness—you just have a strained gluteus medius muscle, causing a strength deficit that is easy to resolve so that you no longer catch your foot or trip so often.

NO CANE FOR YOU!

Assistive devices have concerned me for a long time, particularly in terms of the decay in functional quality of life. What does the traditional medical establishment give a person as part of the acceptance that they are aging? A cane. On the surface, it seems like the logical and humane thing to do. The problem is that when a person uses a cane, a portion of their body weight is supported through the arm and cane. This means that part of the load that was supposed to be exclusively supported through the legs has been taken away. Since the legs are required to absorb less of a load, they will now be used less. This means that the muscles of the legs are going to get weaker. Over time, they will continue to weaken and make you more susceptible to falling. The dependence on the cane is actually growing as the cane is being used for longer periods of time.

Once a fall with a cane occurs, you are deemed too unstable to be assisted by a cane alone. You are then given a walker. While the cane used only one hand to help support the body weight, the walker will use both arms. This means a much higher percentage of the body weight will be supported through the arms, taking away the need of the leg muscles to do the supporting. The lesser use of the leg muscles will lead to greater weakness, making you even more susceptible to falling. Once a fall occurs while using the walker, you will be deemed too unstable to bear weight on your own and you will be placed in a wheelchair.

The only way to reverse the cycle of instability is to identify which muscles are weak or imbalanced and strengthen them through a progressive resistance strength-training program. Making the muscles adapt to greater resistances will help them to become stronger and increase mass, eventually reaching a point where you can achieve balance without straining.

KEEP MOVING NO MATTER WHAT

If you are in pain and seek medical attention, what is typically the first suggestion you receive? *Rest.* Although this seems to be a logical answer, it is only a rational one if you understand which tissue is creating the pain. Let's say you had an incident where you twisted your ankle, and pain and swelling developed. This is a time where rest is appropriate. The strained ligament needs to heal. You actually want the inflammatory response to be allowed to occur so that the healing that develops as part of the inflammatory response can continue uninhibited.

Let's say that you had a heart attack, and some type of treatment was performed on the heart. This is a good time to rest. The trauma of the heart attack and subsequent treatment has put stress on the heart, and resting allows healing to occur.

Or let's say that you cut yourself. Treatment can be performed to address the injury. And once treatment is provided, rest is a good approach to allow for the skin to heal.

But let's talk about pain at the neck, back, or extremities. In more than 95 percent of cases that I have treated, the cause has been muscular.

If a muscle strains and elicits pain, the false thought is that an inflammatory response has occurred. Pain and inflammation are often seen as the same thing by the traditional medical establishment. Physicians will suggest that time is needed to allow inflammation to resolve when you feel pain, even if they determine the tissue eliciting the pain is muscle. The general principle is that regardless of the tissue eliciting pain, pain is the result of inflammation and inflammation requires time to heal. Unless swelling, heat, and redness are present along with the pain, then inflammation is not present. Therefore, the idea of waiting to address a muscular deficit is not a logical response.

If the cause of the pain is a strained muscle, the body will perceive that the muscle might tear and will respond by changing the fluid in the muscle into a gluey type of substance. This "glue" will bind the muscle fiber together and prevent it from reaching its optimal length or creating its optimal force, thereby preventing it from tearing. The only way to prevent this process from occurring over and over again is to change the equation of force requirement and force output, which is to say that you must strengthen the straining muscles until the force output of the muscle is greater than the force requirement of the activities being performed.

If you choose the road of resting after a muscle strain has occurred, you are feeding into the cause of the strain. Resting will only allow muscles to weaken further due to disuse, which will widen the gap between the force requirement of the activities performed and the force output of the muscles performing the activities. The muscles will become more susceptible to straining and move you further away from resolving the cause of the pain. I have treated patients a day or two after traumatic events when it was clear that the symptoms were the result of muscular causes. I was able to return these people to full function and full resolution of symptoms in a short period of time because I understood which tissue was responsible and knew that the quicker I could get the muscles back to optimal force output, the quicker the person could have full function without symptom.

Clearly depending on the tissue, rest can be warranted, but in many cases, rest can lead to further presentation of symptoms. The key to knowing when rest is appropriate and when you should keep moving is identifying what tissue has been injured. If the tissue in question is muscular, barring a tear that would require surgery, establish which muscles have been strained and start strengthening them with the appropriate resistance.

YOU'RE YOUNGER THAN YOU THINK

Most people measure their age by the chronological presentation of the years they have been on earth. For many, the mind-set about what can be accomplished or what is suitable to do is based on their chronological age. Certainly the concept of aging as relating to a progressive deterioration of the systems of the body is well founded. The only aspect that I disagree with is the idea that it is linear and uncontrollable.

The time when we imagine granny or grandpa on the porch in a rocking chair waiting for the grim reaper to make his appearance is over. It is clear that people are living longer, more active lives. Thirty years ago, older people focused on end-stage kidney failure and stroke. Now the primary issue that seniors focus on is how to remain independent in their daily life. The shift has moved from systemic deficits to orthopedic ones. Fitness has become less about keeping the heart and lungs working and more about keeping your muscles strong so you can continue to perform daily practical activities.

Likewise, the perception about what older people should be doing is shifting. Seniors are playing golf or tennis deep into their 90s. From a personal perspective, my father, who is in his 80s, plays golf, tennis, or works out every day. It is thrilling to know that he is so fit and can do all that he chooses, including traveling on a frequent basis. People are even working longer, sometimes well into their 80s, because they love to do it and there is no longer a stigma about working beyond retirement age.

Here is the best news about this shift and your ability to control how long you stay independent: muscle is the one tissue that is not affected by the aging process. Whereas the skin, intestines, lungs, kidneys, and other organs have connective tissue in them that can cause loss of function with age, muscle has an innate contractile force, even while resting.

There are people who perform strength training deep into their 80s and 90s. These people are astounded that they are stronger than they were in their 30s and 40s. They are training their muscles to adapt to greater resistance, which causes their muscles to grow and become stronger, resulting in greater ease and less chance of injury while performing activities.

Don't let your age determine what you do. Let your physical capacity determine it. Incorporate strength training into your lifestyle, and you will be able to do things you couldn't do when you were a lot younger.

AGING DOESN'T MEAN BEING INFIRMED

Another false mind-set that has crept into our culture over the years is that aging and infirmity go hand in hand, where we see getting sick as part of the aging process. However, I feel this attitude is changing due to the facts that people are living longer and that the focus with regard to systemic disease has shifted to sustaining independence.

The best thing a person can do is stay active using the parts of the body that were designed to allow this to occur. And I am not just talking about the muscles and bones. Muscles and bones require energy to work and oxygen to exist. The body requires an immune system to keep you safe. All the nutrients, oxygen, and cells that keep you safe need to be transported around the body via the circulatory system.

All of your body's systems are stressed in a controlled manor, which means they have to work harder when you are active rather than if you are still. This is not an excessive stress that can lead to injury. It is a controlled stress that leads systems and their muscles to become more efficient in how they work. The four elements that lead to good health and prevent illness are:

1. Performing strength training

2. Getting the right nutrients

3. Achieving proper sleep

4. Keeping stress at a minimum

Getting the right nutrients allows the muscles to perform optimally. Ensuring the right amount of sleep gives the body the chance to heal properly and prevents disease from anchoring itself into the different bodily systems. Keeping stress at a minimum reduces an overworking of the neurological system and minimizes the force output of muscles that tend to increase tone during stress. And of course, incorporating regular strength training such as the Yass Method into your regular routine will keep your muscles strong and supple, enabling you to enjoy an active life.

I have met way too many people who felt that being sick is a natural part of getting older. They felt there was nothing they could do to control the illnesses that befell them. They didn't see the connection between being infirmed and having pain, even when the pain was due to muscular causes.

Don't get caught up in the idea that aging means illness. Strength train, eat well, get the right sleep, and minimize your stress so you can be healthy and, most importantly, enjoy your life.

CHAPTER EIGHT

You're on Your Way to a Better Life

RESOLVE PAIN FOR LIFE

The Yass Method not only addresses your pain now, but it also allows you to understand the cause of your pain at any time in the future. Pain is a part of the body's emergency defense system. It is your body's way of trying to let you know when something isn't working correctly. When you have a kidney stone, you get pain at the lower back. If you have pneumonia, you feel upper back pain. The very symptoms you experience when something is not working are being broadcast by the tissues that are in distress.

Why would a muscle, bone, or nerve be any different? That is what the Yass Method is all about: interpreting the symptoms that the body presents to identify which tissues are in distress. The Yass Method works from the head to the foot. It doesn't matter what part of the body you are talking about. If you are trying to establish which tissue is eliciting symptoms, the best way to identify that tissue is by interpreting the symptoms being presented.

The Yass Method has the ability to answer all the questions that don't seem to be able to be answered by the existing traditional model of diagnostic tests. It is based on scientific forces, biomechanics, and the ways in which muscles work to create activity. The Yass Method recognizes that the reason most people suffer from chronic pain is because we live in a gravity environment, meaning that a force is being imposed on us every time we want to perform a task. The group of muscles responsible for creating that task must then create a force equal to that of the force being applied to us. If all the muscles involved in performing the task are not strong enough, one will strain. This can elicit pain or cause other muscles to try to compensate, which leads them to also strain and elicit pain.

Using this method, I have helped to resolve the symptoms of people from age 6 to 102. I have helped to resolve the pain of people who have had multiple surgeries and yet still had the same if not greater pain after the surgeries. Those addicted to prescription pain medication have used the Yass Method to resolve chronic pain. And I have helped to resolve the pain of people who have suffered for up to 40 years with their pain. The Yass Method has the capacity to identify the cause of your pain regardless of your circumstances and at any time in your life.

TUNE UP, DON'T GIVE UP!

It is critical for you to realize that the chronic pain you are experiencing is not of your own doing, nor are you making up the pain in your mind. After treating people who have had pain destroy their lives, I can tell you that nobody chooses to or pretends to be like this.

When you go to specialists, they have no choice but to see your symptoms as somehow falling into their particular specialty. Just think how vast the body is and how a specialist is only trained and educated in one system. The most logical approach to establishing the cause of pain is to look at many possible causes.

Knowledge is indeed power. I want you to have the most knowledge possible so you can understand why you may still be in chronic pain after all your attempts to resolve it.

You will have to make a decision about how you want to move forward in your treatment. You will have to be your best advocate. You will have to ask questions and do the things that feel right for you. I want everyone to have their pain resolved. And it is my hope that the Yass Method helps you to find the cause of your pain and the right treatment for it.

Appendix

The Exercises

In this section I have gathered all the exercises I have recommended in previous chapters so that they are in one place for easy reference. After each exercise's name, I have included an additional descriptive phrase of the general movement involved in the exercise in terms that might be more familiar to you. The list of exercises is presented with the upper body exercises first and the lower body exercises second. Both the strengthening and stretching exercises needed to resolve your dysfunction and resolve your pain are presented.

This is not a book you will simply use one time and put on the shelf. Life has a way of leading to pain at different locations of the body with different activities that you perform at different times. So you may find yourself referencing different sections of this book. Or you might find that you need the strengthening exercises and stretches to resolve pain associated with one particular activity. It seemed to make sense to provide the exercises both where I am discussing the cause of pain from a particular activity, as well as to have them located in one place for easy reference. The key here is that the Yass Method allows a connection to be made between the inability to perform an activity and the pain or other symptoms associated with the dysfunction. Muscular deficit is that connection. Strengthening and stretching the right muscles is the key to achieving an active, healthy, pain-free lifestyle. Embrace the Yass Method and make it a part of your daily life.

STRENGTHENING EXERCISES

Upper Body

➤ **External Rotation:** *Reverse Hammering*

Strengthens the rotator cuff

Means of resistance: dumbbell or resistance band

With the elbow supported at the end of a surface or on a doorknob so that the elbow is just below shoulder height, maintain the elbow at a 90-degree angle through the whole motion. The elbow of the arm performing the exercise should be in a line with both shoulders (if the elbow is in front of this line, the rotator cuff will have difficulty performing the exercise). The start position is with the forearm facing about 20 degrees below parallel to the ground. The resistance is pulled upward until the forearm is facing about 20 degrees above parallel. Then return to the start position. Keep the range of motion as described. Excessive motion can lead to the rotator cuff straining.

start	finish	start	finish

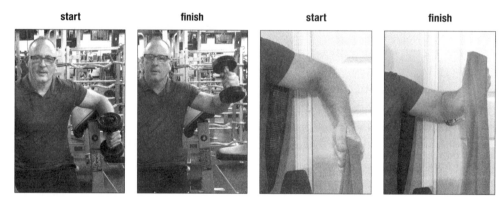

➤ Internal Rotation: *Hammering*

Strengthens the pecs, lats, and teres major and lengthens the rotator cuff

Means of resistance: cable system or resistance band

With the elbow supported at the end of a surface so that the elbow is just below shoulder height, the elbow should be maintained at a 90-degree angle through the whole motion. The elbow of the arm performing the exercise should be in line with both shoulders (if the elbow is in front of this line, the rotator cuff will have difficulty performing the exercise). The start position is with the forearm facing about 20 degrees above parallel. The resistance is pulled downward until the forearm is facing about 20 degrees below parallel. Then return to the start position. Keep the range of motion as described. There is a tendency to go through too much range of motion, which can cause the rotator cuff to strain.

start	finish	start	finish

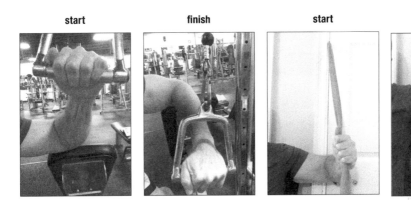

➤ **Lat Pulldown with Neutral Bar:** *Pull Down from Shelf*

Strengthens the interscapular muscles: mid-traps and rhomboids

Means of resistance: Neutral bar or elastic band

Leaning back with an angle at the hip of about 30 degrees (if sitting in a chair, have your butt halfway to the front of the chair while your shoulders are leaning against the seat back), reach up for the bar or elastic band so that the start position begins with your arms nearly straight and your elbows just unlocked. Your feet should be flat on the floor in front of you. Pull the mechanism down, keeping your elbows at shoulder height until your elbows reach just behind the line of your shoulders. The forearms should be maintained in a continuous line with the resistance. Then return to the start position. Don't let your elbows fall during the motion. This will cause you to work a different muscle than the muscles between the shoulder blades.

start	finish	start	finish

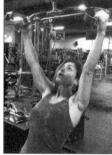 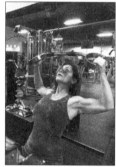 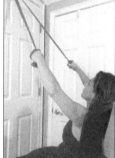 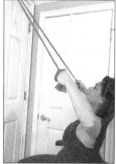

➤ **Lower Trap:** *Paint the Wall*

Strengthens the lower trapezius muscle

Means of resistance: dumbbell or resistance band

This exercise is critical to achieving complete functional capacity of the shoulder. Sit in a sturdy chair and lean back slightly with your butt halfway toward the front of the chair and your back resting against the seat back. If you have difficulty supporting your head while performing this exercise, place the chair against a wall so you can support your head against the wall to prevent the resistance from pulling you forward. Start with your arm halfway between pointing straight forward and pointing straight to the side, with your hand at eye level and your elbow just unlocked. Your palm will be facing in as you grab the resistance. Begin to raise the resistance until the upper arm is in line with the cheek. Then return to the start position at shoulder height. I like to describe this as moving from eye to cheek. Keep in mind that the muscle creating the motion that appears to be occurring at the shoulder is actually at the lower thoracic region and pulling your shoulder blade down your back, which ultimately causes the arm to rise at the shoulder. Try to imagine your shoulder blade being pulled down your back or have somebody put their hand on your shoulder blade so you can feel your shoulder blade moving down the back.

start **finish** **start** **finish**

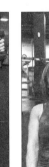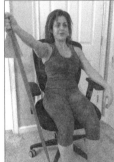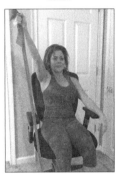

➤ **Posterior Deltoids:** *Gorilla Arms*

Strengthens the posterior deltoids

Means of resistance: dumbbells or resistance band

Stand with your feet more than shoulder width apart, knees slightly bent, and your butt pushed behind you so that you are bending forward slightly. Your weight should be mostly on your heels. Hold the resistance in front of your thighs with your palms facing in and your elbows unlocked (if using resistance bands or tubes, your arms will be at the side of your legs, touching them to start the exercise). Begin to move the resistance out to your side from the shoulders like a pendulum. Go out until you feel your shoulder blades start to move inward (about 60 degrees), and then return to the beginning position.

start　　　　finish　　　　finish (side view)　　　　start　　　　finish

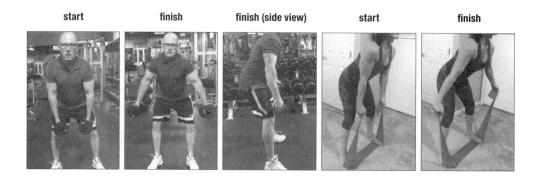

➤ **Protraction Punch:** *Punching with Elbow Straight*

Strengthens the serratus anterior

Means of resistance: dumbbells or resistance band

Lying on your back with your feet supported on the floor, raise the arm performing the exercise so the hand and resistance are directly over the shoulder, with the elbow just unlocked. Then raise the arm slightly using a slow punching movement. This will raise your shoulder slightly off the surface you are lying on (if using resistance band or tube, sit in a chair with your feet planted on the floor in front of you and your back to the door; your arm should be at shoulder height so that you "punch" away from the door). Make sure you do not rotate your torso to try to get more range of motion. Your back should not move at all during this exercise; only the shoulder should rise from the surface. Once the appropriate distance is reached, slowly return to the start position.

start　　　　　　finish　　　　　　finish (close-up)

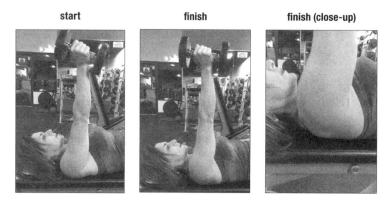

start   finish

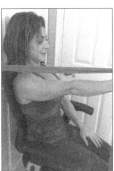 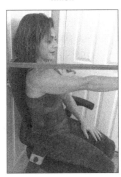

➤ **Tricep Extensions:** *Casting a Fishing Rod*

Strengthens the triceps, single and both arms

Means of resistance: dumbbells, EZ curl bar, or resistance band

This exercise is the most effective way to strengthen the triceps because it puts the long head of the triceps in the optimal position. The long head of the triceps is the only part of the triceps muscle that passes the shoulder joint. Therefore, it is the only part of the muscle that can affect the position of the arm bone in the shoulder joint. This exercise can be performed with one arm or both, depending on whether your pain is associated with one side or requires both arms to be strengthened to resolve it. To perform the exercise, lie on your back with your feet supported on the floor. Start with your arms pointing straight up over the shoulders, with your elbows just unlocked. Keeping your upper arms in place, begin to bend your elbows, lowering your forearms so your hands and resistance are moving toward your forehead. Once your elbows reach 90 degrees, return to the start position. Make sure not to lock the elbows at the top of the motion. (If performing the exercise with a resistance band or tube, sit in a chair with your back to the door and your back supported by the back rest with your feet on the floor in front of you. The resistance band should be set between the door and frame just above head height, and your elbow should be at shoulder height. Grab the resistance band with your elbow at a 90-degree angle and with the palm facing inward, straighten your elbow, keeping the upper arm level until just before the elbow locks. Then return to the start position.)

start	finish	start	finish

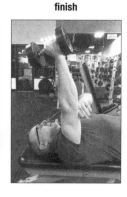 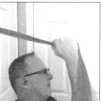 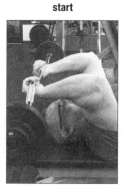 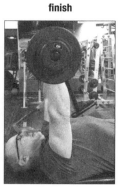

start	finish

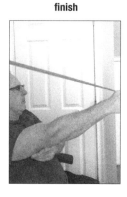

➤ **Wrist Extension:** *Raising Back of Hand*

Strengthens the forearm extensors

Means of resistance: dumbbell or resistance band

Place the forearm on the leg with the wrist hanging in front of the knee and the palm facing down. Place the opposite hand on the top of the forearm to keep it stable and prevent it from raising during the exercise. Start with the hand face down. Bend the wrist upward raising the hand as high as it can go. Then return to the start position.

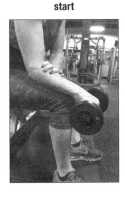
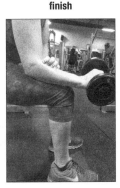
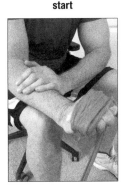
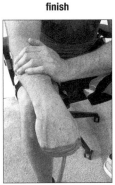

| start | finish | start | finish |

Lower Body

➤ **Dorsiflexion:** *Reverse Gas Pedal*

Strengthens the anterior tibialis

Means of resistance: machine or resistance band

With the leg supported on a surface and the ankle and foot hanging off, attach the resistance so that it is supported in the mid-foot region at the instep. Then attach the resistance between the door and frame near the bottom. You should be seated on a chair and your lower leg supported on another chair or ottoman. The key is that the foot is positioned above the height of the attachment of the band into the door to allow it to remain on the instep throughout the exercise. Start with the ankle angled about 30 degrees forward; then pull the ankle toward the face, about 10 degrees beyond perpendicular. Then return to the start position.

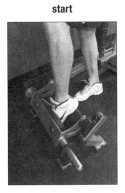
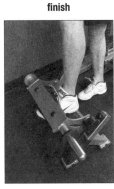
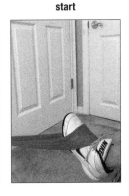
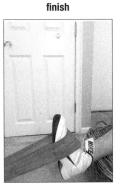

| start | finish | start | finish |

➤ Hamstring Curl: *Reverse Kick*

Strengthens the hamstrings

MEANS OF RESISTANCE: machine or resistance band

In a seated position, place the resistance at the back of the ankle. Make sure you are supported in the seat (if you are using a machine, your lower back should be against the seat back; if you are using a resistance band/tube, position your butt about halfway to the front of the chair while you lean back with your shoulders supported by the chair back). Point your leg straight out with the knee unlocked. Bend the knee until it reaches 90 degrees. Then return to the start position. To isolate the hamstrings better, point the toes of the exercising leg toward your face as the exercise is being performed. In the case of using a seated hamstring curl machine, make sure the pivot point of the machine is aligned with the knee joint. If using a resistance band/tube, there may be a tendency for the knee to rise as the knee is bent. This is because the hamstrings are weak and the body is trying to compensate by using the hip flexors. To prevent this from occurring, place the hand on the same side of the body as the exercising leg on your knee as the exercise is performed. Prevent the knee from rising so that the foot just passes over the floor as the knee reaches 90 degrees of bend.

| start | finish | start | finish |

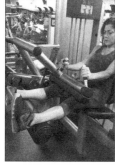 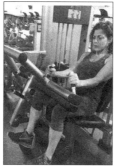 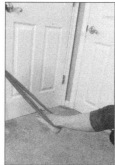 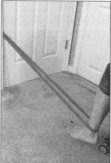

➤ Hip Abduction: *Side Step*

Strengthens the gluteus medius

Means of resistance: cable machine or resistance band

Hip abductions can be performed either lying on your side or standing. To do this exercise correctly, make sure you do not move your leg too far outward. There may be a false sense that more range of motion is better, but in this case, too much range of motion means you are using the lower back muscle to create the motion, not the gluteus medius (hip muscle). The gluteus medius muscle can only move the leg out to the point where the outer portion of the ankle is in line with the outer portion of the hip joint. Any outward motion beyond that is created by the lower back muscle. To do the exercise, lie on your side with the knee of the bottom leg bent and the top leg straight. The top leg should run in a continuous line from the torso. If the leg is angled in front of the torso, you are using a different muscle than the gluteus medius. Start to raise the top leg off the supporting leg until your leg is parallel with the floor. Try to turn the leg in slightly so the heel is the first part of the foot that is moving. This puts the gluteus medius in the optimal position to raise the leg. Once your leg reaches parallel to the floor, begin to lower back onto the supporting leg.

If performing this exercise standing, start with the feet together with the resistance connected to the ankle. Turn the working leg's foot in slightly so the heel is the first part of the foot to move to the side. Step out to the side until the outer portion of the ankle meets the outer portion of the hip. Place this foot on the floor and weight bear fully on it, taking the load off the other foot. Then return the foot back to the start position next to the other foot. Make sure that when you move the working foot out to the side that you are pushing yourself over with the foot you are weight bearing on. Focus your attention on moving the exercised leg over. You may be very weak and feel that you require arm support to perform the exercise correctly. You can place a chair in front of you with the chair back facing you so that you can hold on to it with your hands. The key is not to use this to support yourself beyond what is required.

start	finish	start	finish

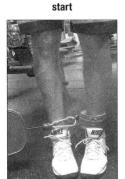 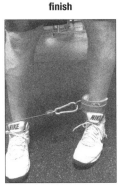 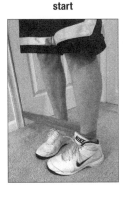 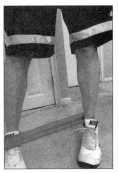

<table>
<tr><td align="center">start</td><td align="center">finish</td><td align="center">finish (side view)</td></tr>
</table>

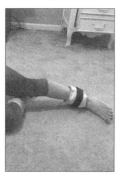 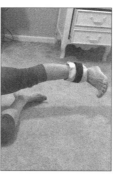 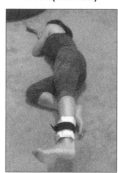

➤ **Hip Extension:** *Kick Back*

Strengthens the gluteus maximus

Means of resistance: machine or resistance band

In a standing position, place the resistance between the door and frame at knee height and then behind your knee. Place the standing leg behind you so it causes you to weight bear against the door and wall with both hands. This will make you feel like you are leaning against the door and wall more than standing on one leg, which will help you to kick behind you without trying to move your body with the leg that is moving. Take the leg that is exercising and bend the knee to 90 degrees. Point the toes forward so the heel leads the foot moving backward. The knee of the working leg should be at least six inches in front of the standing leg's knee at the start. Start to kick behind you until the thigh of the moving leg is in line with the thigh of the standing leg. Then return to the start position. The key to this exercise is for there to be no lateral motion of the body or bending forward and back of the torso. The only thing moving should be the working thigh. Try to keep your back rounded or at least flat so you do not arch the lower back during any part of the exercise.

<table>
<tr><td align="center">start</td><td align="center">finish</td><td align="center">start</td><td align="center">finish</td></tr>
</table>

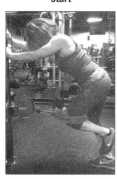 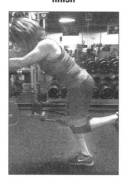 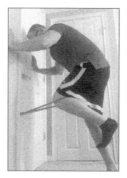 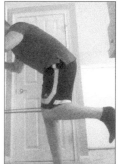

➤ **Inversion:** *Turn Foot In*

Strengthens the posterior tibialis

Means of resistance: cable machine or resistance band

Sitting in a chair, have the resistance coming from your side of the leg to be exercised (if using a resistance band/tube, place the resistance between the door and frame near the floor). Place the resistance around the instep of the foot. The heel should be on the floor with the rest of the foot above the floor. Start with the toes outside the heel and slowly pull the toes in until they are on the inside of the heel. The foot will turn upward slightly as the foot is moved inward. Then return to the start position. Place your hand on the side of the knee of the working leg and make sure it does not move. You do not want any movement or rotation of the working leg. The only motion that should be occurring is at the ankle.

start	finish	start	finish

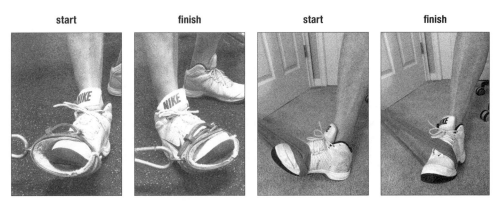

➤ **Knee Extension:** *Seated Kick*

Strengthens the quads

Means of resistance: machine or resistance band

In a seated position, place the resistance around the front of the ankle. Make sure the foot of the opposite leg is on the floor and you are supported in a seat. Begin with the knee bent to 90 degrees, then straighten the knee until it is almost locked. Then return the leg to the start position. Make sure the thigh of the leg that is being exercised remains on the seat and does not rise with the lower leg. If performing with a resistance band/tube, place the resistance under the front leg of the chair next to the working leg. Make sure you make a small loop with the band/tube because you are going to want resistance immediately upon performing the motion of the exercise.

start	finish	start	finish

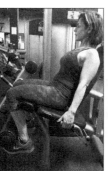 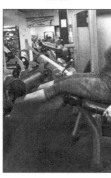 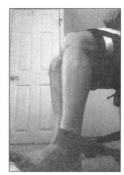 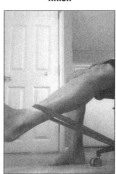

➤ **Leg Press:** *Push Away with Legs*

Strengthens the quads

Means of resistance: machine

When performing this exercise, there is a tendency for the lower back to become rounded as the knees are brought toward the chest. This creates a situation where the spine is no longer supporting the lower back; only the lower back muscles are, which makes them more likely to strain. Only perform the leg press if you have a balance issue preventing you from doing squats or lunges. To do the leg press, place the feet on the plate fairly high so that you are creating a 90-degree angle at the knees and a 90-degree angle at the hips. The plate should not move any farther toward you during the motion of the exercise. Then start to push the plate away from you using your feet with the majority of the force going through the heels. Applying too much force through the balls of the feet means that you will be utilizing a lot of your calves to move the resistance. Move the plate away from you until your knees reach an unlocked position. Then return to the start position. If at all possible, try to keep a slight arch in the lower back during the exercise.

start	finish

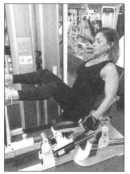 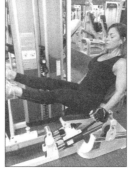

➤ **Lunges:** *Single-Leg Kneel*

Strengthens the quads

Means of resistance: dumbbells or resistance band

Lunges require a bit of balance to complete, so please don't do them if you feel unsteady in any way. You might want to perform this exercise without using extra weight (so you can grab on to something during the motion); however, using resistance in each hand will improve your balance because the weight on either side of your body will help to stabilize you. To do this exercise, spread your feet a little wider than shoulder width apart. Then place one foot in front of you and one foot behind, keeping them the same width apart. The whole foot of the front leg should be on the floor, while only the balls of the foot of the leg behind should be on the floor. Next, lower the back knee toward the floor. The front knee will bend, but make sure it does not end up in front of the front foot. Lower yourself until the front thigh is parallel to the floor. Then return to the start position. Keep the torso upright during the whole motion. The back leg should feel like it is just there for balance. The ability to lower and raise yourself should feel like it is coming from the front foot—that is, you should feel like you are pushing primarily through the heel of the front foot.

start	finish	start	finish

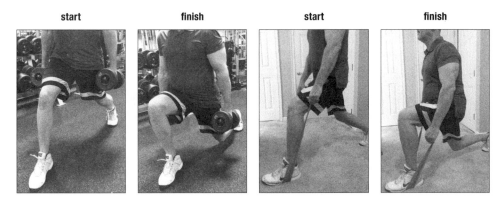

➤ **Sartorius:** *Step One Foot behind the Other*

Lengthens the sartorius muscle

Means of resistance: cable machine or resistance band

Make sure you are holding on to a sturdy object while performing this exercise to help you with your balance. In a standing position, place the resistance around the back of the ankle of the leg to be strengthened. Start with the toes of the leg that is working pointing in slightly. Then place the foot of the exercising leg behind the foot of the leg you are standing on. Once the foot of the exercising leg is placed down on the floor behind the other leg, return it to the start position. Make sure the resistance is appropriate so you can get your exercising foot behind the foot that you are standing on. You want to use a resistance that helps lengthen the sartorius, but because there is a balance element to this exercise, caution should be used in determining the right resistance. Try to keep the knee of the exercising leg straight while the knee of the leg being stood on should be unlocked. Try not to rotate the pelvis as you are performing the exercise. Both the shoulders and pelvis should be facing forward during the whole exercise.

start	finish	start	finish

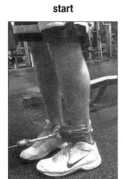 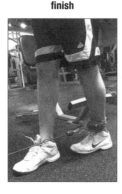 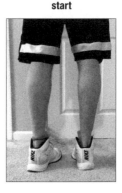 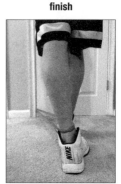

➤ **Squats:** *Sit Down/Stand Back Up*

Strengthens the quads primarily

Means of resistance: dumbbells or resistance band

The main muscle that performs the squat is the quads (front thigh muscle), not the hamstrings or butt muscles. To perform the squat, start with your feet a little more than shoulder width apart and your toes pointed outward. The knees should be unlocked with the butt pushed backward slightly. Hold the resistance in your hands, with your hands at the side of the body. The key to performing a squat properly is to envision that you are sitting down in a chair. The butt should move backward as the shoulders move forward. The knees should remain as close to over the ankles as possible. Remember that a deep knee bend is when you go down and the knee moves forward but the hips stay over the ankles. In a squat the knees stay over the ankles and the butt goes backward as the shoulders move forward. The goal is to sit down far enough until your thighs are parallel to the ground, and then return to the start position. For some, balance might be an issue. If so, don't go too far down. As you gain confidence and strength, you can work your way to the point where your thighs are parallel to the ground. You can also put a chair behind you. This will not only help you visualize the idea of sitting down in a chair; it will also catch you if you lose your balance.

start   finish   start   finish

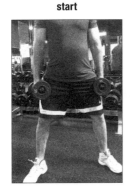 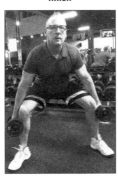 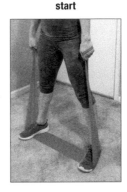 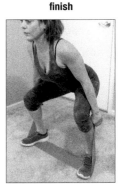

➤ **Standing Calf Raises:** *Come Up on Your Toes*

Strengthens the calves

Means of resistance: dumbbells or resistance band

Start with your feet shoulder width apart, holding the resistance at your side. Bring your heels off the floor, rising up on the balls of your feet (if using a resistance band/tube, place the resistance under the balls of the feet). Then return to the start position. Keep the knees unlocked during the movement. Keep in mind you don't have to raise your heels very far. Just raise them enough to feel like you are balancing on the balls of your feet. If you feel that you have a slight balance issue, place a chair in front of you with the back facing you so you can grab it if you feel unstable.

start   finish   start   finish

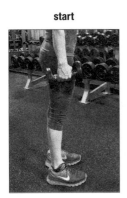 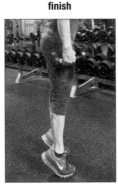 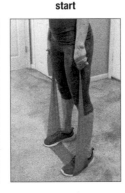 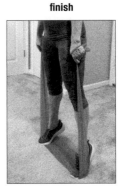

➤ **Straight Leg Deadlifts:** *Run the Hands down the Thighs*

Strengthens the gluteus maximus and hamstrings

Means of resistance: dumbbells or resistance band

Start with your feet a little more than shoulder width apart and your toes pointing slightly out. You should be standing straight with your knees unlocked and your butt pushed back slightly. Hold the resistance in front of your thighs. Bend from the hips, keeping your back straight while looking out in front of you, and begin to lower the resistance down your legs. Make sure your knees don't bend and the motion is coming from your hips. As you move down, you should feel your weight shift to your heels. When you begin to feel tightness at the back of your thighs, slowly straighten back up to the start position. There is no specific point to reach down on the leg. Reach down until you feel tightness at the back of your thighs. Make sure your back remains straight, not rounded. If it's rounded, you can strain your back and you will also go down farther than you could with a straight back. As you go down, you will feel your weight shift back onto your heels. Make sure that the resistance is held tight to your thighs throughout the whole exercise.

start	finish	start	finish

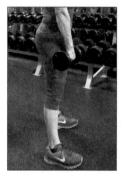 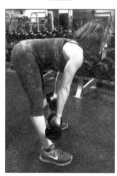 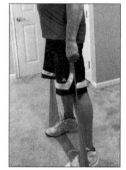 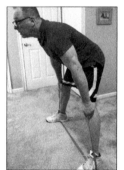

STRETCHING EXERCISES

➤ Calf Stretch

Stretches the calf

Means of resistance: none

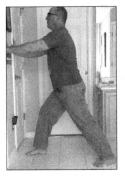

Stand in front of a wall. With your arms straight, place your hands on the wall. Keeping your feet hip width apart, bend one knee and step slightly back with your other foot. The calf of the back leg will be stretched. Make sure the whole foot stays on the floor during the stretch. Keeping the knee of the front leg bent, move your torso forward so more of your body weight is on the front leg. Continue moving forward until you feel a stretch in the back calf. Once you feel the stretch, hold it for 20 seconds and return to the start position.

➤ Gracilis Stretch

Stretches the gracilis

Means of resistance: none

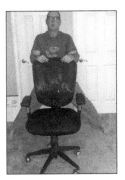

Stand next to a wall or an object that you can use to support yourself. Gradually move your legs out to the side, spreading slowly until you start to feel a stretch at the inner thighs. Make sure your knees are unlocked when performing this action. Hold the stretch for 20 seconds and return to the start position. You may not get very far before you feel a stretch. That is okay. Just continue with the process, and over time you will be able to stretch farther. The key is to perform this stretch slowly, only spreading your legs enough to feel a mild stretch.

➤ Hamstring Stretch

Stretches the hamstrings

Means of resistance: none

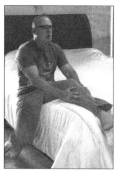

Sitting on a surface with the leg to be stretched pointing in front of you and the other leg hanging off the side, place your hands on the thigh of the leg to be stretched. Make sure your back stays in a straight position and you don't hunch. Start to move your chest toward the leg out in front of you, keeping the knee unlocked and the toes pointing forward, away from your face. Continue to move the chest toward the leg until you feel a stretch at the back of the thigh. Once you feel the stretch, hold it for 20 seconds and return to the start position. You may not go too far before feeling the tightness at the back of the thigh. That's okay; you will improve over time.

➤ Hip Flexor Stretch

Stretches the hip flexors

Means of resistance: none

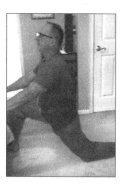

Kneel down on one knee next to an object that will help you balance when performing this exercise, such as a chair or couch. The leg you are kneeling on is the one with the hip flexor that will be stretched. Slowly move the opposite leg in front of you with your other foot on the floor and the knee bent. Begin to move the pelvis forward with your torso upright so you start to move closer to the front foot. You will begin to feel a stretch at the upper thigh region of the leg you are kneeling on. Once a comfortable stretch is felt, hold it for 20 seconds.

➤ ITB Stretch

Stretches the ITB

Means of resistance: none

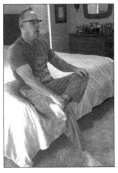

Start by sitting in a chair with both feet on the floor. Place the ankle of the leg you are trying to stretch on the opposite knee. Put both hands on the knee of the leg you are trying to stretch and slowly press the knee down toward the floor, feeling a stretch at the outer thigh anywhere from the hip to the knee. Once a light stretch is felt, hold the position for 20 seconds. Then return to the start position. Your ITB may be too tight to be able to put the ankle on the opposite knee. If this is the case, start by placing the ankle halfway up the shin and holding it there with one hand while pressing down on the knee. This can be progressed until the ankle can finally be placed on the opposite knee to perform the stretch.

➤ Pec Stretch

Stretches the pecs

Means of resistance: none

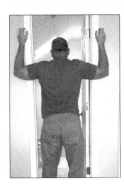

Stand in a doorway with your elbows at shoulder height. For those with long enough arms, the elbows will be sitting on the doorframe. If you have shorter arms, the elbows might be just inside the doorframe. With your feet centered in the doorway, begin to lean forward, keeping the torso upright. Your chest will begin to move slightly in front of the line of the shoulders, creating a pulling sensation at the front of the shoulders where the pecs attach to the shoulders. Move forward enough to create a light stretch. Hold this position for 20 seconds. Then return to the start position and repeat.

➤ Piriformis Stretch

Stretches the piriformis

Means of resistance: none

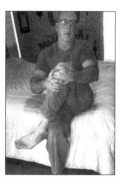

Sitting in a chair with your back supported, place the ankle of the leg to be stretched on the bent knee of the opposite leg. If the ankle cannot be placed on the knee, just place it as high up on the shin as possible. Then with both hands, grab the knee of the leg to be stretched. Pull the knee toward the opposite shoulder until a stretch is felt in the butt. Once you feel the stretch, hold it for 20 seconds and then return to the start position. This stretch can be used to diminish sciatic symptoms for short-term relief.

➤ Quad Stretch

Stretches the quads

Means of resistance: none

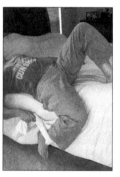

Lie on a surface with the leg to be stretched hanging off the side and the other leg on the surface with the knee bent and the foot on the surface. Next, place a towel around the ankle of the leg to be stretched in order to give you something to hold on to. Grab the towel and slowly begin to bend the knee toward the butt until a stretch is felt in the front of your thigh. Once you feel the stretch, hold it for 20 seconds and return to the start position. Make sure that your back does not arch while performing the stretch. This is a very stable position for stretching the quad and most people should be able to do this (versus the commonly suggested quad stretch of standing up and pulling the heel toward the butt).

Endnotes

Chapter One

1. Maureen C. Jensen et al., "Magnetic Resonance Imaging of the Lumbar Spine in People without Back Pain," *The New England Journal of Medicine* 331 (July 14, 1994): 69–73. http://www.nejm.org/doi/full/10.1056/NEJM199407143310201#t=article.

2. Ibid.

3. W. Brinjikji et al., "Systematic Literature Review of Imaging Features of Spinal Degeneration in Asymptomatic Populations," *American Journal of Neuroradiology* 36, no. 4 (April 2015): 811–816. https://www.ncbi.nlm.nih.gov/pmc/articles/PMC4464797/.

4. Roger Chou et al., "Diagnosis and Treatment of Low Back Pain: A Joint Clinical Practice Guideline from the American College of Physicians and the American Pain Society," *Annals of Internal Medicine* 147, no. 7 (October 2, 2007): 478–491. http://annals.org/aim/article/736814/diagnosis-treatment-low-back-pain-joint-clinical-practice-guideline-from.

5. A. G. Filler et al., "Sciatica of Nondisc Origin and Piriformis Syndrome: Diagnosis by Magnetic Resonance Neurography and Interventional Magnetic Resonance Imaging with Outcome Study of Resulting Treatment," *Journal of Neruosurgery: Spine* 2, no. 2 (February 2005): 99–115. https://www.ncbi.nlm.nih.gov/pubmed/15739520

6. Baber, Zafeer, and Michael A Erdek. "Failed back surgery syndrome: current perspectives." *Journal of Pain Research*, Dove Medical Press, 2016, www.ncbi.nlm.nih.gov/pmc/articles/PMC5106227/.

Index

Note: For specific exercises, page numbers in *italics* indicate explanations of how to perform the exercises, and page numbers in normal font indicate other routines incorporating them.

C

D

E

F

K

L

M

T

Acknowledgments

To Reid Tracy and Patty Gift, for having the courage and confidence to print this book, I thank them. Millions will benefit from the contents within and it is only through their leadership that this information is being made available so widespread.

To Lisa Cheng and Annie Nichol, thank you for taking my science-based and sometimes "highly technical" information and making it understandable. The greatest information in the world has little value if it cannot be understood by the masses and you both helped to make this possible.

To my wife, Lisa, and my daughter, Natalya, there are not enough words to explain your impact on my life. I feel blessed that I was given this ability to see things in a unique way that helps people live the types of lives they choose. All the rest of my thought and soul go to you for making each day so special.

About the Author

Dr. Mitchell Yass has spent the past 25 years developing his method of diagnosing and treating the cause, not the symptom, of pain. His unique Yass Method is based on carefully interpreting the patients' symptoms instead of relying on diagnostic tests. He has helped many thousands of patients resolve their pain and thousands of others avoid unnecessary surgery. Dr. Yass believes that his effective, noninvasive methodology should be the standard of care provided to patients suffering with pain rather than the traditional, expensive, and often-ineffective treatments including MRIs, pain medication, and surgery.

When Dr. Yass is not providing care, he enjoys weight lifting, golf, and spending time with his wife and daughter. Dr. Yass received a doctorate in physical therapy from the New York Institute of Technology and is the author of *The Pain Cure Rx* and *Overpower Pain*. You can visit him online at www.mitchellyass.com.

Hay House Titles of Related Interest

YOU CAN HEAL YOUR LIFE, the movie, starring Louise Hay & Friends
(available as a 1-DVD program, an expanded 2-DVD set,
and an online streaming video)
Learn more at www.hayhouse.com/louise-movie

THE SHIFT, the movie, starring Dr. Wayne W. Dyer
(available as a 1-DVD program, an expanded 2-DVD set,
and an online streaming video)
Learn more at www.hayhouse.com/the-shift-movie

———

*YOUNG AND SLIM FOR LIFE: 10 Essential Steps to Achieve Total Vitality
and Kick-Start Weight Loss That Lasts,* by Frank Lipman, M.D.

THE 3 CHOICES: Simple Practices to Transform Pain Into Power, by Jorge Cruise

All of the above are available at your local bookstore,
or may be ordered by contacting Hay House.

———

We hope you enjoyed this Hay House book. If you'd like to receive
our online catalog featuring additional information on Hay House
books and products, or if you'd like to find out more about the
Hay Foundation, please contact:

Hay House, Inc., P.O. Box 5100, Carlsbad, CA 92018-5100
(760) 431-7695 or (800) 654-5126
(760) 431-6948 (fax) or (800) 650-5115 (fax)
www.hayhouse.com® • www.hayfoundation.org

———

Published in Australia by:
Hay House Australia Pty. Ltd., 18/36 Ralph St., Alexandria NSW 2015
Phone: 612-9669-4299 • *Fax:* 612-9669-4144 • www.hayhouse.com.au

Published in the United Kingdom by:
Hay House UK, Ltd., Astley House, 33 Notting Hill Gate, London W11 3JQ
Phone: 44-20-3675-2450 • *Fax:* 44-20-3675-2451 • www.hayhouse.co.uk

Published in India by: Hay House Publishers India,
Muskaan Complex, Plot No. 3, B-2, Vasant Kunj, New Delhi 110 070
Phone: 91-11-4176-1620 • *Fax:* 91-11-4176-1630 • www.hayhouse.co.in

———

Access New Knowledge.
Anytime. Anywhere.

Learn and evolve at your own pace
with the world's leading experts.

www.hayhouseU.com

Free e-newsletters from Hay House, the Ultimate Resource for Inspiration

Be the first to know about Hay House's free downloads, special offers, giveaways, contests, and more!

 Get exclusive excerpts from our latest releases and videos from *Hay House Present Moments*.

 Our *Digital Products Newsletter* is the perfect way to stay up-to-date on our latest discounted eBooks, featured mobile apps, and Live Online and On Demand events.

 Learn with real benefits! *HayHouseU.com* is your source for the most innovative online courses from the world's leading personal growth experts. Be the first to know about new online courses and to receive exclusive discounts.

 Enjoy uplifting personal stories, how-to articles, and healing advice, along with videos and empowering quotes, within *Heal Your Life*.

 Have an inspirational story to tell and a passion for writing? Sharpen your writing skills with insider tips from *Your Writing Life*.

Sign Up Now!

Get inspired, educate yourself, get a complimentary gift, and share the wisdom!

Visit www.hayhouse.com/newsletters to sign up today!

 HAY HOUSE

 HAYHOUSE RADIO
radio for your soul

 HAYHOUSE
online learning

Tune In to *Hay House Radio—* *Radio for Your Soul*

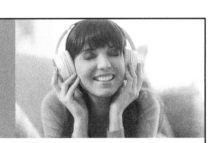

HAY HOUSE RADIO offers inspirational and personalized advice from our best-selling authors, including Anthony William, Dr. Christiane Northrup, Doreen Virtue, James Van Praagh, and many more!

Enjoy **FREE** access to life-changing audio 24/7 on HayHouseRadio.com, and with the Hay House Radio mobile app.

Listen anytime to the Hay House Radio archives of over 13,000 episodes (and more added daily!) with a Hay House Radio All Access Pass.

Learn more at www.HayHouseRadio.com